Move for Life

Move *for* Life

A Practical Guide to Building Everyday Strength, Balance, and Confidence for *Thriving After 65*

Damien A. Joyner
Foreword by Dr. Evan Osar

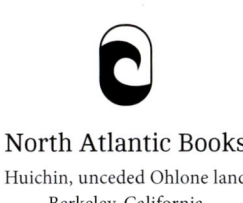

North Atlantic Books
Huichin, unceded Ohlone land
Berkeley, California

North Atlantic Books
Huichin, unceded Ohlone land
2526 Martin Luther King Jr Way
Berkeley, CA 94704 USA
www.northatlanticbooks.com

Cover art © SpicyTruffel via Getty Images
Cover design by Jasmine Hromjak
Photos by Minivan Productions
Book design by Happenstance Type-O-Rama
Printed in the United States of America

Move for Life: A Practical Guide to Building Everyday Strength, Balance, and Confidence for Thriving After 65 is sponsored and published by North Atlantic Books, an educational nonprofit that collaborates with partners to develop cross-cultural perspectives; nurture holistic views of art, science, the humanities, and healing; and seed personal and global transformation by publishing work on the relationship of body, spirit, and nature.

North Atlantic Books's publications are distributed to the US trade and internationally by Penguin Random House Publisher Services. For further information, visit our website at www.northatlanticbooks.com.

The authorized representative in the EU for product safety and compliance is Eucomply OÜ, Pärnu mnt 139b-14, 11317 Tallinn, Estonia, hello@eucompliancepartner.com, +33757690241.

PLEASE NOTE: The creators and publishers of this book disclaim any liabilities for loss in connection with following any of the practices, exercises, and advice contained herein. To reduce the chance of injury or any other harm, the reader should consult a professional before undertaking this or any other movement, health, or exercise program. The instructions and advice printed in this book are not in any way intended as a substitute for medical, mental, or emotional counseling with a licensed physician or healthcare provider.

Library of Congress Cataloging-in-Publication Data

Names: Joyner, Damien A., 1978- author
Title: Move for life : a practical guide to building everyday strength, balance, and confidence for thriving after 65 / Damien A. Joyner ; foreword by Dr. Evan Osar.
Description: Berkeley, California : North Atlantic Books, [2025] | Includes bibliographical references and index. | Summary: "A Practical Guide to Building Everyday Strength, Balance, and Confidence for Thriving after 65"-- Provided by publisher.
Identifiers: LCCN 2025000413 (print) | LCCN 2025000414 (ebook) | ISBN 9798889842811 paperback | ISBN 9798889842828 epub
Subjects: LCSH: Self-actualization (Psychology) in old age | Older people--Conduct of life | Older people--Health and hygiene | Older people--Psychology
Classification: LCC BF724.85.S45 J69 2025 (print) | LCC BF724.85.S45 (ebook) | DDC 155.67--dc23/eng/20250625
LC record available at https://lccn.loc.gov/2025000413
LC ebook record available at https://lccn.loc.gov/2025000414

1 2 3 4 5 6 7 8 9 Versa 30 29 28 27 26 25

To the diverse community of active agers.

*Know that you are seen and deserve to
reap the benefits of exercise so you can keep
a firm grip on your independence.*

CONTENTS

FOREWORD

Because of chronic tightness or pain, too many of us are unable to live the life we want. One of the most fundamental keys to maintaining longevity, independence, and feeling full of life is physical activity. Since most of us don't get enough physical activity, we must strategically include exercise in our daily routine. In his book, *Move for Life*, Damien outlines a simple foundation for living the life you want while feeling great in the process. Furthermore, Damien provides real-world examples of how applying the right type of training can help you in virtually every aspect in your life. Whether your goal is to walk longer without having to stop, work in your garden without back pain limiting you, hike a mountain, or beat your friends at pickleball, this book is for you. *Move for Life* bridges the gap between where you are now and living your life with the energy, strength, and endurance you need to accomplish your goals.

Dr. Evan Osar, author of *Corrective Exercise Solutions
to Common Hip and Shoulder Dysfunction*

ACKNOWLEDGMENTS

I extend my deepest gratitude to my parents, Al and Corrine Joyner, for your unwavering support and inspiration. I feel fortunate to have been raised in a loving household where healthy meals are made from scratch, the value of helping others is instilled through example, and laughter is always in abundant supply. Special thanks to my parents and my big brother, Quincy, for always being in my cheering section—even when you sometimes wondered what the heck I was doing.

To my close friends and mentors who have believed in me through thick and thin, I am profoundly grateful for your support. I appreciate the time you spent reminding me I was overthinking things, asking me probing questions, and offering your shoulders to lean on when I felt stuck. You know who you are. You know what my journey to discovering my purpose has entailed. Man, we have some stories, don't we? Much love to all of you.

I would like to thank every client I have worked with. You have enabled me to grow both professionally and personally. Your resilience, commitment, trust in me with your emotions and fears (and your body!), and effort in the gym inspire me every single day.

To my friends at the American Council on Exercise (ACE), thank you for trusting me with so many opportunities for professional and personal growth. I am immensely grateful for all of it.

My sincere thanks to everyone at North Atlantic Books—my acquisitions editor, copyeditors, proofreaders, design team, indexer, creative director, and print production manager. Your dedication and expertise have elevated my dream of a published book beyond what I envisioned. I also extend my appreciation to Kyler Beal, Lead Storyteller of Minivan Productions, and to our models—Martha Ranson, Debra Bass, Ruth Johns, and Dr. Anthony Biascan—for their generous help with the photographs.

And thank you, dear reader, for picking up this book and taking the time to read it. I trust you will find useful nuggets of information and inspiration to guide you on your fitness journey.

INTRODUCTION

The population of older adults in America is growing steadily. According to 2023 census data, more than fifty-nine million people aged sixty-five and above live in the United States.[1] You are part of a diverse group that is living longer than ever before and cannot be pigeonholed into a single way of living or one set of interests. However, there is one thing you all have in common: the desire to maintain the ability to do what you need and want to do in life.

Your generation leads varied lives. Each of you has unique family and work responsibilities that keep you busy. For some, there are opportunities to travel and explore after retirement. You have lived through substantial technological and societal changes, like the invention of wearable fitness trackers, virtual personal training, cell phones, and webinars on countless topics. You continue to leave your mark on society through work, volunteering, and legacies you have built. Whether choosing to work longer or have more time to enjoy retirement, your generation has more opportunities to live life on your terms than any previous one. However, there is a significant problem.

Part of the problem is a lack of support and advocacy for older adults to be more physically active. The key to addressing this issue is shifting how the fitness industry treats older individuals—recognizing that you have the potential to learn, improve, and discover new ways to move your body. Because you do! Unfortunately, our society often perpetuates the idea that life is "over" at a certain age, a mindset that is reflected in the fitness industry and beyond. Prescribing only gentle exercises for older adults creates a self-fulfilling prophecy. This kind of guidance does not equip people to navigate a world that requires strength, power, agility, and balance to move in. If you can walk into a gym, limiting you to seated exercises is unreasonable. If you have knee or hip issues, there are safe and effective ways to improve mobility and strength. Promoting the idea that certain exercises should never be done after fifty[*] focuses solely on the individual's age, dismissing their fitness level and potential. This systemic ageism, when internalized or expressed, increases the risk of becoming part of the alarming statistics on rising rates of falls and chronic health problems among older adults. Ageism can negatively affect how exercise is prescribed or recommended, leading to overly cautious or inappropriate advice. The form or intensity of a movement should be tailored to your physical abilities, not your age.

The other part of the problem is that many older adults are not moving as much as they should. Why do people tend to exercise less, or stop exercising altogether, as they get older? Some reasons for this are common across all ages: lack of time, finding exercise boring, or fear of injury. Pain, particularly chronic pain, is another significant factor. It can reduce motivation to engage in any activity that might worsen discomfort, including certain types of movement. Additionally, some individuals internalize the ageism prevalent in our society, believing they should stick to gentle exercises and avoid strength training entirely. However, avoiding exercise for these reasons creates a harmful cycle—a negative feedback loop that leads to a self-fulfilling prophecy. Reduced activity can result in frailty, loss of independence due to difficulty performing daily activities, and greater susceptibility to falls.

To address the lack of movement among older adults, we must become part of the rising tide that empowers them to be strong, agile, flexible, confident, and independent. Many fitness professionals, researchers, organizations, and healthcare professionals are already leading this charge, but self-advocacy is just as important.

Don't be part of the problem; don't let your age be an excuse for what you believe you can't do. You can still enjoy physical challenges through exercise, enhancing your quality of life. You can learn more optimal ways to move, whether on your own or with the guidance of a personal trainer. Yes, exercise today may look different than in your twenties or thirties, but you can—and should—still strength train in your fifties, sixties, seventies, and beyond. The

---

[*] You may have come across a social media post sharing a *Reader's Digest* article titled "14 Exercises to Never Do After Age 50." The claims made in that article are completely false, and the original article has since been removed. If you did happen to read it, I strongly advise against following its recommendations.

drive to exercise should be even stronger and more urgent as you age because it is vital to maintaining independence and confidence.

This book serves as your roadmap to staying active as you age. Even if the word *exercise* doesn't resonate with you, practicing movement in ways that challenge you can reduce your risk of falls, boost your confidence, and improve your quality of life.

Put simply, the solution is to practice movement that helps you function better in your everyday life. To remain active, there are things you *must* move and do. Granted, what makes life exciting are the things you *want* to do. But if you can't move with ease to get out of a chair, pick something up off the floor, or get down and back up again, how can you do the things you want, like plan a trip to a national park, play with your grandkids, or give back to your community?

Use this book to inspire you to move more and be more independent. Use it to break out of your usual routine and try a group exercise class. Use it to justify investing in a personal trainer who has experience working with active agers and can challenge you safely. If this book was a gift, it means someone cares deeply about your quality of life—and that, in itself, is a gift.

A QUICK NOTE ABOUT NUTRITION

This book focuses on exercise, but a good quality of life also includes healthy eating habits. The benefits of a balanced diet include fat loss, muscle growth, and a reduced risk of chronic diseases. Since I am not a nutritionist, providing specific dietary advice is beyond my scope. However, the general advice I give to all my clients is to stay hydrated by drinking water, eat plenty of veggies, cook meals from scratch, get sufficient protein, and limit sugar intake.

As you might be aware, nutrition advice is everywhere you turn and often accompanied by mixed messages about what to eat or avoid. Many of my clients find it helpful to explore cookbooks or online recipe resources, which can also make healthy eating more enjoyable. Others benefit from personalized guidance. For tailored advice, I recommend consulting a qualified nutritionist or dietitian—someone who can focus on your unique needs and goals.

Why You Can Trust Me to Guide You: My Journey and Philosophy

As the founder and owner of Incremental Fitness™, I specialize in helping active agers move better and improve their quality of life. Early in my journey in the fitness industry, I discovered how much I enjoy working with this demographic. What I love most about my work are those exciting lightbulb moments when clients realize the connection between what they do in the gym and how it helps them in their daily lives. These moments help clients understand why I challenge them in the gym—so everyday activities can become less of a challenge.

During my time as a fitness professional, I have noticed a significant lack of space for older adults in the industry. Fortunately, there is hope as the environment is becoming more inclusive. Organizations like the American Council on Exercise (ACE) are leading this shift by equipping fitness professionals with the knowledge and resources necessary to work effectively with active agers. I earned my Personal Training Certification from ACE in 2016 when I began my career in fitness. Since then, I have been actively engaged with them and currently serve as a subject matter expert (SME) on their Certification Advisory Board and Virtual Certification Committee. In this role, I have also represented ACE in various media publications, been featured in their video study materials and marketing campaigns, and contributed to educational efforts by developing and leading the webinar "Exercise Strategies for Clients with Physically Demanding Jobs." This webinar is now available to fitness professionals for continuing education credit. Beyond ACE, I have been certified as a Functional Aging Specialist through the Functional Aging Institute (FAI), which has greatly shaped my expertise. FAI's study materials ensure that exercise options accommodate all fitness levels while addressing both the physical and cognitive benefits of exercise. My work is further informed by my certification as an Integrative Corrective Exercise Instructor from the Integrative Movement Institute (IMI). Dr. Evan Osar and his team at IMI provide fitness professionals with tools, classes, workshops, and certifications that teach how to help clients find more optimal ways to move and breathe, both in the gym and in daily life, even when facing challenges such as chronic pain or joint issues.

Thanks to my background in the nonprofit sector and the importance of giving back instilled in me as a child, I approach my work with empathy and a desire to help. I recognize that our emotions are closely tied to our ability to move. I see and feel the frustration that clients experience when they struggle with new movements or realize they can no longer do something they once could. My experience has taught me that taking the time to explain the benefits of an exercise, pausing a workout for a pep talk, and celebrating small victories all make a big difference in clients' progress. I have learned to first listen—both to what a person is saying and not saying—before determining how I can best support them. From leading group classes in San Diego for over twenty active agers to working one-on-one with clients of all ages, I have honed my ability to meet clients where they are.

My law school education also contributes to my approach. I tend to analyze movement closely when observing clients exercise, always looking for ways to make the connection between exercise and everyday life as clear as possible. Often, this connection is vague or underemphasized in broader discussions about fitness, perhaps because exercise is typically framed around how we feel while working out, with little attention given to how it benefits our lives outside the gym. Simply telling someone that exercise is good for them often goes unheeded. I believe that helping them see the real-life benefits of exercising makes it more tangible and increases their buy-in. This is why I prioritize learning how my clients regularly spend their time outside of training. This understanding allows me to create stronger connections between their activities in the gym and their everyday lives, enabling me to tailor training that is relevant and impactful.

Exercise Prepares You for Your *Game Day*

Let's look at this through another lens: sports.[†] What is one of the main things you want for the players you support, aside from winning? You want the athletes to stay off the injured list as much as possible. When an athlete is healthy and uninjured, they can effectively compete. How do they ensure they remain injury-free? They train for their sport. Athletes must always be physically

---

[†]   Bear with me—I am not a big sports enthusiast. My good friend Shomari calls me a "closeted sports fan" because, while I do enjoy watching the Holiday Bowl, some tennis, and track and field, I can easily frustrate a sports fan with my limited knowledge of current games and indifference to whether a team wins or loses. I just enjoy watching a good game . . . sometimes.

prepared for the demands of their game. If a player slacks off during the off-season and underperforms during practice, how much confidence would you have in them on game day?

Everyday life involves movement, so every day is like game day for you. We should all move in ways that prepare us for the demands of daily living. Continuing with the sports analogy, what happens if a player gets hurt? They are not simply sent home to sit on the couch and watch TV all day. Recovery for athletes involves rest, but it also includes rehab and a structured exercise regimen to get them back in the game. Going from the couch to game day takes preparation and consistency.

This aspect of training and preparation applies to you and ties directly into the title of this book. You want to live a life of joy, prosperity, and independence for as long as possible. The key to longevity will not be found in a bottle of pills, cortisone shots, or some celebrity-endorsed fad. Being mindful about nutrition, addressing chronic disease, and taking preventative measures can all contribute to longevity. At the same time, movement is an absolute necessity. Movement is what makes life truly worth living. When we think about a loss of independence, one of the first things that comes to mind is the inability to walk, clothe, feed, or bathe ourselves. When someone struggles with everyday activities, it not only affects their independence but also takes a toll on their mental health and overall outlook on life.

Getting on the Proactive Path

Later in this book, I discuss the graph in figure 1 in more detail. For now, let's focus on the two paths it illustrates and how they diverge. As you transition to the "Older Age" life stage, the disability threshold does not have to be part of your future. By disability, I mean the inability to perform the everyday activities essential for independent living without assistance from others. Sitting on the couch, eating poorly, neglecting exercise, and not finding ways to move better can set someone on the trajectory represented by the lower line. This book is about staying on the upper line for as long as possible. Even if you find yourself nearing or at the disability threshold, there are still opportunities to move better!

The only way to ensure movement remains not a challenge, or becomes less so, is through physical challenges. You may not be heading to the squat rack to perform a loaded squat with a barbell and one hundred pounds on

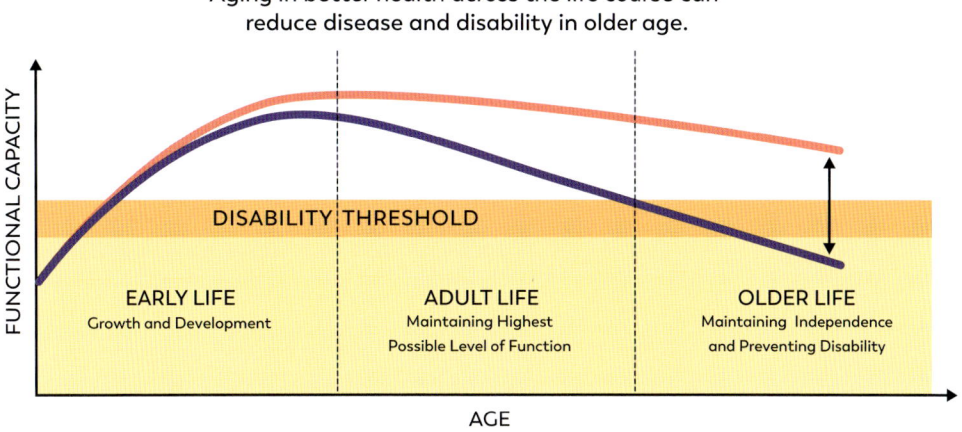

Source: Adapted from Kalache, A., Kickbush, I. A Global Strategy for Healthy Aging. *World Health*, 1997 50(4)-S.

FIGURE 1. Functional capacity and the aging process. Adapted from an original work published in *World Health*, a journal by the World Health Organization[2] (Creative Commons, CC BY-NC-SA 3.0 IGO).

your back, but you can improve at getting out of a chair. You may not be cranking out one hundred burpees, but you should be able to get down to the floor and back up again. Carrying groceries, moving objects, and bending over are all activities you should be able to do comfortably in your daily life. What I want to help you avoid is the tendency to shy away from activities or movements due to decreasing strength, agility, flexibility, or conditioning. Even if you can do everything you want now, what steps are you taking to ensure this remains true as you age?

You need to exercise. While you may not be thrilled by the conventional definition of the word, I am sure you enjoy doing the things that make you happy. Exercise is a vital part of maintaining the ability to do those things. Be vigilant about addressing chronic diseases as well as hearing and vision issues, as these also play a role in your overall independence. A great article by Baylor University's MPH online program discusses a 2018 study[3] revealing that "48 percent of physicians and nurse practitioners routinely failed to recommend exercise when advising older patients about falls."[4] Don't assume your doctors will bring up exercise—it is up to you to make it a priority. A consistent exercise routine helps maintain or improve strength and balance, both of which reduce the risk of falls.

Need more compelling statistics? The same article cites findings that "27% of adults aged 45–79 reported at least one fall in the past 12 months, according to a 2014 study. 11% reported an injurious fall, meaning it resulted in activity limitation or healthcare utilization. 25,180 people aged 75 or older died from a fall in 2016, compared with 8,613 in 2000, a 192% increase."[5] These numbers underscore the connection between falls, hospitalizations, and fatalities associated with falls. Balance training, strength training, and agility training can help reduce the risk of falls. These exercises promote increased confidence in movement and improve reaction times, enhancing your ability to catch yourself from a potential fall. The more you find ways to safely challenge your balance and train for fall prevention, the better your outcomes will be.

Finally, I want to leave you with some words and phrases that resonate with my rockstar clients—individuals who embrace the importance of exercise.

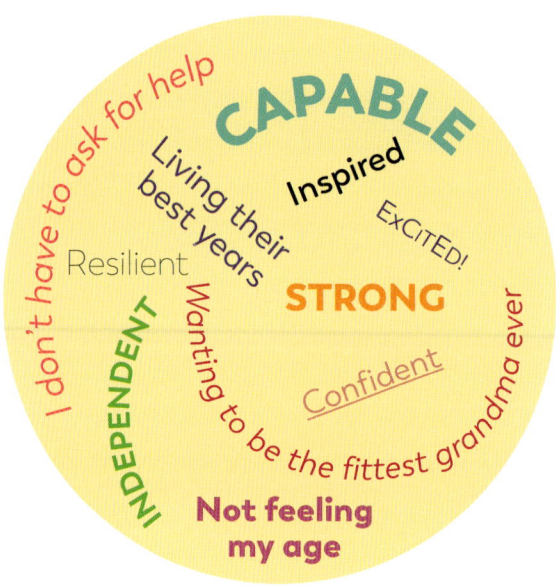

FIGURE 2.

All these words and expressions can be part of your vocabulary too. I believe you deserve the respect of being challenged so that everyday life can be less of a challenge. The joy of movement isn't reserved for the young—it's for everyone.

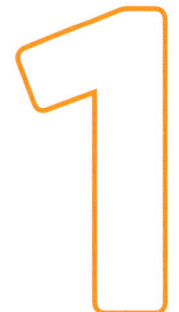

THE JOY OF MOVEMENT

We do not so much quit playing because we grow old,
as grow old because we quit playing.

—GEORGE L. KNAPP, "ANCIENT ORIGIN OF MODERN SPORT,"
IN *THE OREGON JOURNAL*

When we were children, we engaged in a lot of learning—not just in school, but also by exploring the world around us and learning how to move within it. This stimulating process included crawling, reaching, touching things, and figuring out how to stand and walk. As adults, we often find joy in seeing children go through this process and watching their little lightbulb moments as they discover something new.

For a more eloquent explanation of this stage of life, let's turn to Sally Goddard Blythe, director of the Institute for Neuro-Physiological Psychology. In her book *The Well-Balanced Child: Movement and Early Learning*, she writes:

A child gains its first experience of the outside world through movement. During the first 9–12 months of life, the infant will acquire thousands of new movement patterns and movement abilities. At the same time as these movements are being learnt, the infant replicates the brain development of its evolutionary ancestors, passing from the aqueous environment of the womb where movements were fish-like in character, to crawling on its belly like a reptile creeping in hands and knees like a mammal, "cruising" on two feet whilst using the hands for support, and eventually gaining confidence and control of balance on two feet.[1]

You may be wondering why I am focusing on the nature of movement during our younger years. One reason is that fitness professionals often look back to these developmental stages of our lives for reference. During our early years, we generally experience movement without many of the restrictions, tightness, or injuries that adults often face. Think about a toddler sitting in a deep squat position, casually playing. How many adults do you know who can sit in that position comfortably? During this stage, learning and making mistakes are accepted, understood, and expected. This perspective is vital: Striving for perfection should not be the goal of exercise. Instead, the goal should be practicing and improving.

It is also important to connect our movement patterns as children with those we use as adults. I want to underscore that the foundational movement patterns Blythe describes, which we first acquire as children, are the same ones we constantly rely on as adults. These movement patterns include:

- pulling things
- pushing things
- getting down on the ground and getting back up again
- sitting down and standing up (aka, squats)
- picking things up and putting them somewhere

These patterns are integral to how we move every day. They are also the movements that fitness professionals, like me, encourage you to practice. There is never a point in life when you should stop improving your movement patterns. Period. Never stop. Especially if you currently face restrictions in how you move, be vigilant. The more you practice, the more you learn how to move better. This can reduce your risk of injury and chronic disease while keeping a hold on your independence. The benefits of moving better extend beyond how good you look; they also relate to functionality. When I say *vigilant*, I don't mean you should force a square peg into a round hole—avoid painful movements. If how you perform squats consistently hurts your knees, pause and seek advice about your form instead of pushing through the pain. Let go of the idea that you must strive for perfection when learning new movements. Instead, focus on improvement and progress toward your goals. You will learn at your own pace through setbacks and successes. Allow yourself to grow without judgment.

Let's take a closer look at how these foundational movement patterns show up in our daily lives:

- getting out of bed

- going to the bathroom

- dressing and bathing yourself

- picking up unevenly weighted objects and moving or placing them elsewhere

- lifting a pet or child and placing them down

- navigating uneven, slippery, or varied surfaces

- getting in and out of a car

- performing movements required for your job or hobbies

- reaching overhead or down low to retrieve items

While these tasks and movements might seem boring or mundane, they are fundamental to maintaining independence and a good quality of life. In the fitness industry, these movements are referred to as "functional." Functional exercises mirror daily life movements and can help you perform all the aforementioned actions with greater ease and confidence. For example, let's consider the functional exercise of squats and how it translates to the everyday activity of using the bathroom. Sitting down on a toilet involves balance and leg strength to not only sit down but also descend slowly to avoid crashing down. When standing up, you push off with firmly planted feet to rise to an upright position. Ideally, you should be able to perform both sitting and standing movements without using your hands for support. This is similar to how the squat is commonly performed at the gym, often with an external weight held in the hands. However, variations can be introduced that allow you to use your arms for support while still working on building leg strength.

Now that we understand how foundational movements relate to our daily life, let's connect this to the title and theme of this chapter: joy. What are your favorite activities? What movements do they require? Consider experiences like vacations, playing with your grandkids, golfing, dancing, or going to the movies. Every activity that brings us joy involves movement. The foundational movement patterns we engage in every day—often without thinking about them—enable us to do the things that make us happy.

We often focus solely on the enjoyable moment or activity without acknowledging the preparation and movements that led up to it and made it possible. In the same way that quality ingredients contribute to an amazing meal, foundational movements make our fun and memorable moments possible. For this reason, I want to break down the physical steps required to do the things that bring us joy.

Breaking Down Everyday Movements

Let's break down an activity—having a friend over for dinner—into its component movements to illustrate how movement is interwoven into our lives. Even if you don't or can't cook, you can in this scenario! You're welcome.

1. **Morning routine.** You wake up and carry out your morning routine, which includes getting out of bed, going to the bathroom, showering, and getting dressed. These actions require balance, leg strength, arm and core strength, and flexibility.

2. **Traveling.** Next, you head to the store or farmers market. Whatever mode of transportation you use requires physical effort, but for this example, let's assume you are driving. You must be able to get into your car and move your neck to check the mirrors. Exiting the car also involves certain movements like shifting your weight to stand on one foot, balancing momentarily, and stepping out.

3. **Shopping.** At the store, you grab a cart, push it, and walk around. You may encounter stairs, escalators, or ramps and navigate them. The items you select for dinner are on shelves at various heights, requiring you to reach high or squat low to access what you need. You may twist your body to place items into your cart. As your cart fills up and gets heavier, you push with more effort. If you are carrying your groceries in a basket or bag instead, you will engage your balance, agility, single-arm strength, single-leg strength, and core strength to move around. All these movements happen naturally while you shop and may feel mundane when they are not challenging. However, when any of these movements become difficult, you suddenly become acutely aware of the effort involved.

4. **Loading your groceries.** You lift and place your groceries into your vehicle. Even if your car isn't high off the ground, this task requires balance,

core strength, pulling, and some pushing. As you leave the parking lot, you again navigate curbs, concrete parking blocks, and whatever obstacles Mother Nature may be throwing your way. When you are walking with your loaded grocery bags, you are carrying unevenly distributed weight in your hands or on your back.

5. **Unpacking at home.** Once you get home, the groceries won't unpack themselves! Unloading your vehicle involves nearly the same movements as loading it, but in reverse, along with the added challenge of navigating your home's terrain.

6. **Putting groceries away.** If you are more organized than I am, you'll put everything where it belongs instead of piling it on the counter. This requires lifting items off the ground and putting them away on shelves, either high or low. Handling the individual items can also call for hand dexterity and grip strength.

Finally, you sit down to enjoy the amazing dinner you've prepared for your friend. The effort was well worth it, and it took physical activity to make it happen.

Better Movement Does Not Stop at the Gym

In a gym or similar setting, we often focus on form and progress. Both are subjective to the individual. In this controlled environment, people with varying goals practice better movement. When you return to your everyday life after a workout session, it is important to continue using the tools you learned in the gym. Going back to the dinner example: While preparing a meal, you pick things up and move them around your kitchen. At the gym, you do similar actions—picking things up and moving them. The form and technique you practice in the gym should carry over into your daily activities, like cooking.

Remain mindful of your movement throughout the day, not just during workout sessions. Even if you have an amazing personal trainer or group class leader to guide you a few hours a week, this still applies. Continuing movement outside the gym can be as simple as practicing better squat form when sitting down or lifting something off the ground in a safer way. It is up to you to decide how best to incorporate better movement into your life in a way that suits your routine and needs.

This connection between better movement and life outside of however you exercise is critical to realize. At the gym, I see my clients, and others' clients, accomplish impressive things. That is awesome. Yet, the most impressive part is how those accomplishments translate to their daily lives. One of the best parts of my job is hearing clients share what they can now do, or do better, in their everyday life. Using your body to climb stairs at a national monument or step into a boat to go sailing embodies what, in my eyes, better movement is all about.

Let's face it: The average person who exercises is not always stoked about every workout. However, they are excited about what they can achieve with their body because of those sessions and their dedication.

Move as much as you can during the day. Find ways to move outside your scheduled workouts. The more you move, the stronger the connection becomes between your structured exercise time and recreational time where you are active without even thinking about working out. Here are some examples of how you can incorporate movement outside your scheduled exercise time:

- Choose a parking spot farther from the entrance to add a longer walk to and from your car.

- Take the stairs instead of the elevator or escalator.

- Walk and sit tall. Don't slouch.

- Stand up and walk around regularly, especially if you have been sitting for long periods.

- Opt for a spirited walk instead of a slow stroll.

- Practice standing up from a chair without using your hands.

Build a Strong Foundation

Your foundation consists of all the activities you perform in your everyday life. These include getting up from a chair while holding something, gardening tasks, stepping onto a curb, or placing luggage into an overhead compartment. These everyday movements are not rigid or confined to a gym environment, which is why people often don't recognize how these actions mirror gym exercises. For example, gym exercises like pressing or pulling directly translate to actions such as pushing a wheelbarrow, lifting yourself out of bed, or pulling a rake. There is a clear connection.

When it comes to fitness, we tend to focus on measurable goals: how much we can lift; the number of repetitions, or *reps*, we can complete; how many steps we take in a day; our weight; doing an impressive new exercise; or achieving a new personal best. While these numbers can be great motivators and help to track progress, I encourage you to also recognize what can't be quantified—like how you feel. There is no metric for confidence, but we all understand how moving with greater confidence can improve our outlook and sense of well-being. Similarly, though we cannot measure balance improvement in numbers, there is a peace of mind that comes from walking without anxiety about falling.

Your foundation is not only broad but also deep, encompassing multiple layers of movement. Let's illustrate this with a short fictional scenario: Meet Sam. Sam can push an impressive amount of weight on the leg press machine. She consistently incorporates strength training for her legs into her workouts. However, Sam is not doing any balance training and has noticed that her balance is not as good as it used to be. She decides to just "be careful" when walking to avoid falling.

It is natural to enjoy doing what we are good at, and balance training often falls off the radar, even for vigilant active agers. However, simply being careful won't help Sam improve her balance; in fact, avoiding activities that challenge her balance could lead to further limitations. Instead, Sam should work on improving her balance just as she has worked on her leg strength. If she wants to improve her balance but doesn't know where to begin, someone like me can introduce her to exercises that enhance and solidify foundational movements.

Think of all the different kinds of movement that support our everyday life activities. These movements form our foundation and serve as crucial building blocks. If we are unable to perform them, the things we need and want to do become significantly harder. This foundation includes:

- balancing
- walking and navigating obstacles
- lifting
- pulling
- pushing
- eye-hand coordination

Movement Pyramid

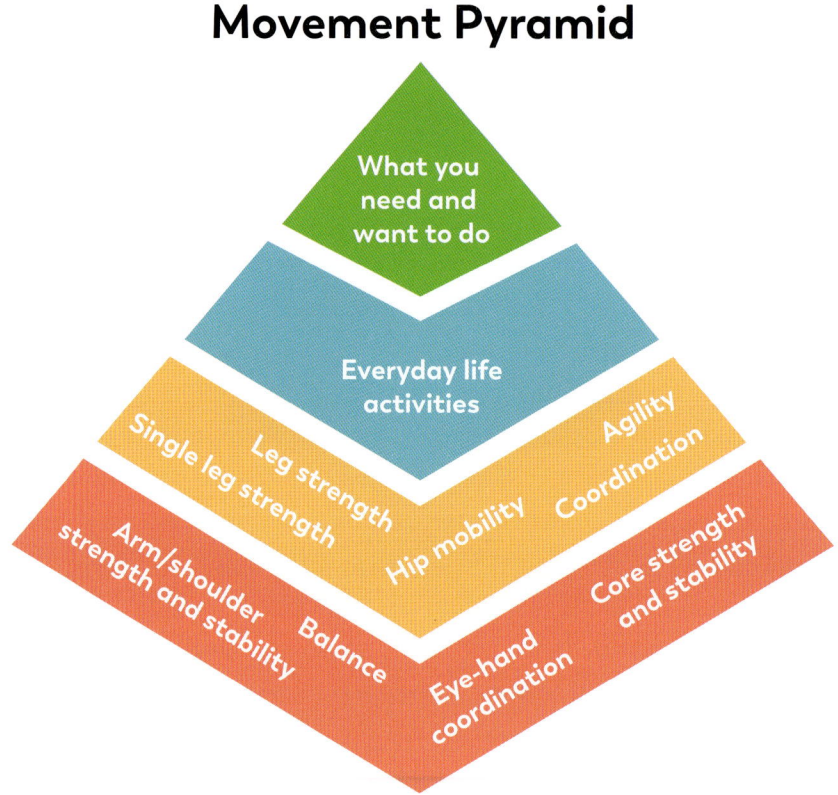

FIGURE 1.1.

- body awareness (knowing where your body is in space and moving it without consciously focusing on each individual movement in relation to your surroundings)
- stability to move objects or yourself with control

These movements may seem insignificant to those of us who perform them effortlessly, but they can profoundly impact our quality of life. It can be sobering when foundational movements like walking or sitting become challenging.

I encourage you to notice and appreciate these small movements, even on your worst days. Keep challenging yourself, and allow others to challenge you to move better in life. Celebrate the little movements you make as you wake up each morning, and ensure they remain second nature. You do this by finding ways to safely challenge yourself, so these movements continue to feel easy. Regardless of your age, exercise—in its many forms—enables you to keep doing what you want and love in life.

Start Where You Are: Own Your Movement Journey

Original Strength (OS) is a dedicated group of individuals who generously share their knowledge of movement to help people reconnect with their bodies, increase mobility, and move better. They offer certifications and training not only for fitness professionals but also for individuals who want to learn and benefit from improved movement. Many of their ideas resonate with me, and I incorporate them into my work with clients.

In their certification booklet, OS provides a valuable perspective on movement that I want to share:

> Any movement is good. If movement can be made, change can take place. Every individual has their own starting point. They have their own physical history, their own structure, their own capabilities, and their own current limitations. However they move is good.[2]

What I want you to take from this is that your journey begins at the "You Are Here" point on your map. Your *good* may not be the same as mine or anyone else's, and that does not matter. What matters is what you can do today. Starting where you are physically allows you to accept how you move right now. It is okay if your current abilities are not where you want them to be. If you struggle with squats but can sit in an elevated chair and stand back up, then that is your *good*. Acknowledge that inactivity or skipping your essential (but sometimes mundane!) physical therapy homework may have led you to your current state. If you feel that you are in great shape and move well, then that is your *good*, and I challenge you to learn how to move even better so you can continue progressing on that path.

Exercise, in its many forms, is often about learning. We learn how to move in specific ways and how our bodies respond to those movements. Broadly speaking, when you work with a personal trainer, they teach you movements tailored to your goals and current abilities. Then, you practice those movements.

When your session is over, your aim should be to "own" the good movements you have practiced. To own a movement is to perform it with control and confidence. For instance, owning a squat means lowering yourself to a safe depth with control, pausing at the bottom, and then returning to a standing position. Whether consciously or subconsciously, you continue to practice these improved movements. Sometimes, these improvements feel subtle, and you may not even notice that you are moving differently or better.

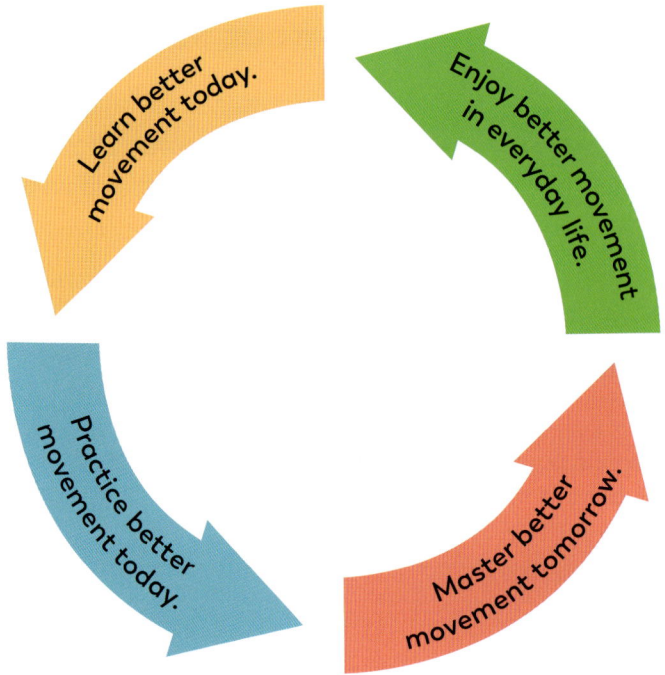

FIGURE 1.2. Movement journey

However, even slight changes in a movement you are being mindful of can have significant benefits. For instance, practicing good posture can reduce the risk of lower back injuries and prevent neck pain by keeping your neck in a more optimal position.

OS also emphasizes the transition from good to better to best. Optimal movement is your best movement. What is optimal for me may not be optimal for you, and that is absolutely fine. Forget about achieving perfection—your optimal movement does not need to be perfect. Instead, focus on moving better each day. Make this a lifelong pursuit, paving the way to the quality of life you deserve.

The Snowball Effect: Better Movement Leads to Better Movement

Moving better in life creates a snowball effect in slow motion—the more you do it, the more you can do over time. If you are just getting back into a movement routine, prioritizing better movement should be your focus. Build and stick to good routines. Incorporate healthy habits, such as being more mindful of what you put in your body and drinking more water. Some soreness is to be expected; it is par for the course. Over time, you will start to notice changes. Sometimes these changes are so gradual that you may not see them right away, but friends and family might. Perhaps your walking stride becomes smoother, you can pick things up off the floor more easily, or you can walk upstairs without needing to use the railing.

Your movement can become easier, more comfortable, and less effortful. But remember: This process takes time. Don't fall for infomercial-style promises. Don't expect overnight results or a thirty-day transformation. Like the common disclaimer says, "Results may vary." Yes, achieving better movement takes effort and focus from you. But along the way, you will experience small wins. Notice them. Celebrate them. Allow yourself to reconnect with your body, and you will see how these small victories add up.

At the time of writing, I have a client who is a very active sixty-nine-year-old. She kayaks, swims, rides a bicycle, and lives life to the fullest. We worked on her balance, and it improved over a few months. As her ability grew, I added new challenges to match her progress. One exercise involved her balancing while having something nearby to hold onto if she became unsteady. Over time, I encouraged her to decide for herself whether she needed the support. Soon, she stopped asking for it. This small win was huge. Not only did it demonstrate her improved balance, but—perhaps more importantly—it reflected her increased confidence.

Now imagine how that confidence and ability snowball into her everyday life. It enhances how she gets into and out of her canoe and boosts her confidence that she can mount and dismount her bicycle more smoothly, even in a pinch. I am not suggesting she's about to join a gymnastics group (though that would be cool!), but she is enjoying more and better-quality movement in the activities she already engages in. With greater confidence and improved movement, you might find yourself trying things you have never done before.

That, my friend, is the joy of movement. You don't need to reach all the way back to your childhood to appreciate the importance of practicing better movement. But as I mentioned at the beginning of this chapter, tapping into that creativity and optimism can inspire you now. Life is not about the impressive feats you can achieve in the gym. It is about how you utilize your body once you leave the gym. You should be enjoying movement with confidence, navigating a three-dimensional world.

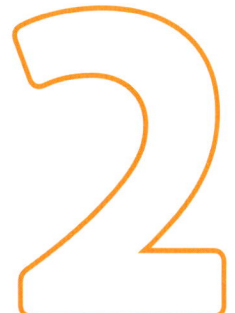

MOVING IN A THREE-DIMENSIONAL WORLD

> *Aging is out of your control. How you handle it, though, is in your hands.*
>
> —DIANE VON FURSTENBERG, *THE WOMAN I WANTED TO BE*

Our world is three-dimensional, with length, breadth, and depth. We navigate this space in various directions, often while holding objects, animals, or children. Even when we move in one direction, our movement is rarely linear. Consider the act of getting into a car. We don't simply sit down; we shift our weight, place a foot or hand into the car, and engage our entire body to get into the seat. This seemingly simple act is actually quite complex. It involves balance, agility, strength, eye-hand coordination, control, and flexibility. On top of that, the surfaces we navigate can vary widely—they may be slippery, uneven, soft, hard, steep, or even covered with seasonal elements like wet leaves or ice.

In this chapter, I will explain how we move in our everyday lives to highlight the importance of practicing better movement. Every movement we make, even when it feels effortless, requires us to account for many factors. Practicing better movement helps us navigate the world, both inside and outside our homes. The ability to move confidently, efficiently, comfortably, and with reduced risk of injury is a true win-win.

We rarely travel in a straight line in our daily lives. Even a simple walk down the street can involve navigating curbs, potholes, or other obstacles that necessitate changes in our direction or movement. We may need to shift our bodies diagonally or laterally to avoid colliding with other pedestrians or to squeeze through narrow spaces. If we don't lift our feet properly, we risk tripping. The inability to pick our feet up—whether to clear a rug, a curb, or an uneven sidewalk—can lead to a fall. Similarly, the objects we lift, move, or carry are rarely as perfectly weighted or convenient to hold as a dumbbell. For instance, a large sack of potatoes lacks handles and does not distribute weight evenly. Even something easy to hold, like a grocery bag, is often carried in one hand, creating uneven strain on the body.

Why is all this important to point out? Our lives involve diverse forms of movement on varied surfaces. Practicing movements that mimic these real-life scenarios helps you move more confidently, comfortably, and safely in your daily life. Let's break it down further.

Navigating a Three-Dimensional World Involves Complex Movement

A lot happens physically when we move in our daily lives. Sitting down in a chair while holding a bag isn't just a squat. Picking up an item and placing it on a shelf isn't as simple as it seems. Walking up the stairs with a bag of groceries is a complex movement. Even the act of walking is intricate. Getting out of bed? That's yet another example of a surprisingly complex movement. Over time, we have become so used to doing all these movements that we take our abilities for granted—until we start to experience difficulties in executing these tasks. Then we might say: *Oh, it's old age.* But I want to challenge that mindset. Movement does not have to be difficult. Your desire to move should be just as strong and urgent as it was when you were a child.

The Surfaces You Move On Are Not All Flat or Uniform

From the moment you get out of bed, you encounter physical obstacles. These include rugs that may shift underfoot, carpet, hardwood floors, and tile floors that can be slippery—especially when wearing socks or footwear with little traction. Then there are stairs, loose gravel, sloping driveways or walkways, and the surprises Mother Nature may have in store outside.

If you live in the city, you will encounter sidewalks and streets that are rarely perfectly flat or free of cracks. Even in a meticulously maintained area, you have to navigate curbs when crossing the street. Stairs, sidewalk cracks, and other uneven surfaces turn walking into an obstacle course with varying levels of difficulty.

The density of the terrain we walk on varies as well. Dirt may feel softer than other surfaces, while loose dirt or rocks make for an unstable surface. Enjoying the outdoors, whether in your local park or a national park, requires navigating inclines, declines, and a variety of terrains. And let's not forget about ice or that white stuff that falls from the sky (I have been in San Diego for so long that I can't quite remember its name)—walking on either of those is vastly different from walking on dry concrete.

Uneven and unstable terrains also affect our speed. We may need to adjust how quickly we move to avoid falling or to navigate obstacles in our path. When walking on loose gravel or slippery ground, we can't pivot or turn as quickly as we might on carpet or solid ground. Finding the sweet spot between balance, stability, agility, and efficient movement toward our destination employs much more than just leg strength.

Nonlinear Movement

Movement in everyday life is rarely a linear path. Our actions don't follow perfect forty-five-degree angles or straight lines. Consider some examples:

- **Getting in and out of a car.** This involves leaning, shifting weight, and turning. Even if your vehicle requires you to step up, you still need to lean to get in.
- **Walking down the street.** While a sidewalk may be relatively straight, curbs still require you to get up and over. Cracks, debris, dog poop, or

other hazards in your way can force you to adjust your steps. Navigating around objects or other people may also necessitate moving quickly to avoid collisions.

- **Picking up and transferring objects.** These tasks involve much more complex movement than a simple lift, twist, and deliver motion. Think about the clunky old-school depiction of robots and their rigid movements. Our bodies, in contrast, move fluidly—often in ways we may not notice until we encounter problems with these once-menial tasks.

The connection I want to highlight is that we don't walk, lift, twist, pivot, or balance in perfectly straight lines. Mundane tasks entail complex movements in environments that call for us to move in various directions.

Better Movement, Better Navigation

Many of the movements we perform daily are variations of lunges and squats. However, I sometimes hear, "Oh, I don't squat or lunge. Those are bad for my knees." A client once expressed this concern during her first session. My response was to remind her and everyone else that if they go to the bathroom, sit down, or pick things up off the floor, they are already doing some form of squats or lunges. Often, a client's concern stems from knee issues, which can lead them to associate specific movements with pain or an inability to perform them.

Let go of the standard you may have in your head. Put aside how you see others performing these movements in workout videos or at your gym. You already engage in variations of squats and lunges every day. You find ways to sit down, stand back up, and pick things up off the ground. Sometimes, you may compensate to accomplish these movements, but you still do them. For example, rocking your body to get out of a chair instead of just standing up is a compensation. You have created your own variation of the movement. Your adaptations may arise from eroded balance, pain, a lack of strength, or other issues. While these variations help you complete tasks, they may contribute to further injury or pain because they involve moving your body in less-than-optimal ways.

However, go easy on yourself; many of these variations are created unconsciously! The good news is that you can learn more optimal ways to move while also gaining strength and reducing pain or discomfort in the process.

For instance, strengthening your core from different angles, combined with practicing deadlifts (a type of weightlifting exercise), can help you pick things up from the ground with less lower back pain. Another byproduct of improved movement is confidence. While confidence isn't easily measured, the ability to move with ease and assurance is invaluable.

The same client who initially avoided lunges and squats eventually worked with me to perform variations that reduced stress on her knees. She did great! She practiced better movement during our sessions, mastered her good movement on her own, and was surprised—and thrilled—by what she could do.

Your everyday life is filled with lunges, squats, and other movements that can be practiced in a gym setting. Practicing these movements in a controlled environment will help you, over time, to carry out everyday tasks with relative ease.

Better Movement at Work and Play

Do you enjoy golf? Are you an avid tennis player? Are there other sports or activities you love doing? Is your work physically demanding? If you answered yes to any of these questions, this chapter will resonate with you. Enjoying activities that require you to move in different directions is all about mastering three-dimensional movement. You might think, "Oh, I'm not that competitive" or "I get enough of a workout from playing or working." However, that mindset could shorten your longevity on the court or in the workplace. Remember, the goal is to avoid injury and maintain good health. This means training in ways that lower your chances of getting hurt on game day.

If you are a tennis player, don't you want to improve your swing and keep it strong? Practicing your swing can benefit your game, but developing core strength is equally important. Are planks enough to improve core strength for tennis? Of course not. Planks are a static exercise, while tennis is a dynamic sport played while standing. There are variations of planks that incorporate movement, but these still don't replicate the standing or half-kneeling positions typical in tennis. Tennis players also benefit from exercises that enhance power and speed, which in turn contribute to improving core strength. Even an activity like bowling, which involves moving in a straight line with weight in your hands, requires you to own each position with strength, stability, and confidence. You may not be the most competitive player, but you likely want to maintain or even improve your skills.

Practicing your sport helps, but cross-training to build a rock-solid move-ment foundation is equally, if not more, essential. Cross-training is one of the best ways to reduce the risk of injury. It will have you moving in different direc-tions than usual, building agility and resilience. Plus, it can be a lot of fun!

Let's say you aren't a sports enthusiast but enjoy gardening. Gardening involves moving in various directions, often on unstable surfaces, to get the job done. Planting, weeding, watering, pulling a stubborn hose, raking, dig-ging holes, and many other gardening tasks require multi-directional move-ment combined with strength, balance, and flexibility. Even if you believe the hours spent working outside count as a workout, incorporating some formal exercise ensures you can continue to dig holes, pull weeds, or squat down to check on your seedlings. Keeping your foundation of movement strong is essential for enjoying your favorite activities for years to come.

If your job involves being on your feet all day or performing manual labor, practicing better movement is critical for doing your job safely. Long hours may leave you feeling like you don't have time to exercise or stretch, but con-sider this: What would happen if you could no longer physically perform your job? The time you invest now to stay fit and healthy is priceless. If you want to enjoy your retirement, don't wait until retirement to start exercising. Exercises you do to strengthen your back today could prevent injuries tomorrow. Being more vigilant about stretching now could mean less tightness after a long week at work. By becoming stronger, you make it easier for yourself to do your job while protecting your ability to work in the long term. Many companies now encourage and even provide resources for employees to exercise during the workday. This convenience allows employees to break up their day with movement that can reduce risk of injury and chronic pain. Investing in your physical health now means you can enjoy both your career and your retire-ment more fully.

Life Involves Complex Movements—Why Not Practice Them?

It is important to recognize that the movements we perform daily are com-plex because they rarely isolate a single set of muscles or joints. While walking into the gym and using the leg press or chest press machines will help increase strength, those exercises do not fully prepare you for the complex movements required in everyday life. For instance, let's say you can do twelve repetitions of 150 lb. on the leg press. Awesome! But ask yourself: Did that exercise test your balance? Did it enhance your core stability and strength? Did it help you move more confidently when stepping to the side? The answer to these questions is no. Similarly, consider the chest press machine. Did it test your single-arm strength and stability? Are you always in a seated position when pushing things in real life? Did it give you the confidence to raise your luggage into the overhead bin? Again, the answer is no.

Everyday movements are dynamic. Getting out of a chair requires leg strength, balance, and stability. Pushing objects and lifting items overhead often involve one hand and arm doing most of the work, while the other stabilizes the object. So, if you're at the gym, why limit yourself to movements or exercises that only work in one direction? To prepare for complex movements, you should practice both simple and complex movements in your exercise routine. Challenge yourself in the gym or work with a qualified professional, so that movements in everyday life become less of a challenge.

Here are some examples to illustrate the difference between simple and complex movements. A basic squat is an example of a simple movement. Some variations to make basic squats more complex include:

- Performing a squat while holding a heavy weighted ball with both hands at sternum level.

- Performing a squat while holding a moderate-weight dumbbell in one hand at your side.

- Squatting to pick up a ball, standing up, and placing the ball on a shelf above your head and to the side.

Don't feel like you need to overthink incorporating such complex movements into your workouts. These variations are meant to help you perform everyday activities that involve movements with varied foot patterns or while carrying external weight.

Why Your Desire to Move Must Be Urgent

Your interest and desire to move should be urgent. I don't mean waking up each day like a sprinter at the starting line and moving as quickly as possible all day long. Instead, take advantage of your ability to move, whenever you can. This means taking the stairs instead of the elevator. It also means taking time to give your body (including your feet!) some TLC through stretching and exercise. Why should the desire to move be urgent? Moving with urgency today will help maintain and improve your ability to move in the long term.

Keeping a firm grip on your independence should be a goal you commit to every day. How you choose to achieve that is up to you. You don't need to run six miles a day, but aim to do more than just walk to the mailbox or take a leisurely stroll on the treadmill. Incorporating exercises that enhance balance, strength, and coordination is crucial for improving or maintaining the quality of life you deserve.

Independence, at its core, is the ability to dress, feed, care for yourself, and carry out everyday activities without assistance. The activities of daily living— like grocery shopping, cooking, and cleaning—form the foundation of our lives. The activities we pursue for fun or work depend upon that foundation.

You have likely seen inspirational stories in the news or on social media about people defying the expectations of their age. These achievements don't happen by accident. People who maintain a high level of independence as they age work for it. They exercise, eat well, drink enough water, take care of themselves, prioritize medical appointments, and address health issues proactively. Some have been consistently active their whole lives. Others were once sedentary but decided to take charge of their health and improve their quality of life. Regardless of their starting point, these individuals invested time and effort to reach a better place. They probably made mistakes, figured out what worked for them, and kept at it. They likely felt bored or dealt with frustration at times—but they kept going. And so can you.

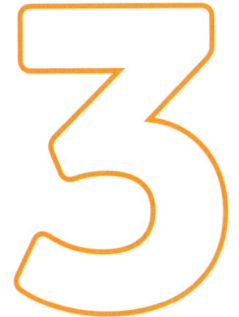

REALLY . . .
HOW FIT DO
I NEED TO BE?

> *We either make ourselves miserable, or we make ourselves strong. The amount of work is the same.*
>
> —CARLOS CASTANEDA, *THE TEACHINGS OF DON JUAN*

At this point, you may be thinking, "Okay Damien, I get it . . . the idea of finding joy in movement and the importance of moving in different directions. But how fit do I actually need to be?" If there were a simple answer to this question, I could give you a mathematical formula where you plug in your age and other factors to get a straightforward response. But you already know it's not that easy. Improving your quality of life and becoming your best version of fit is not about shortcuts. It can be tempting to fall for ads and gimmicks that promise quick fixes, but if something sounds too good to be true, it probably is. Even if such products deliver minor results, they won't solve all your problems. Stay skeptical and do your research. Instead of chasing trends, consider these timeless words widely attributed to the great Arthur Ashe: *To achieve greatness, start where you are, use what you have, do what you can.*

Focus on your own path and stop comparing yourself to others. Everyone faces different physical demands in their daily lives, and physical or cognitive limitations affect what each person can do. Yet, we all share a common need: the ability to perform activities of daily living (ADLs). ADLs include essential tasks, some of which were discussed in the previous chapter, such as picking things up, bathing, dressing, and feeding ourselves. The goal is to minimize the chances of needing assistance with these activities. While assistance may sometimes be unavoidable, such as during illness or when dealing with a restrictive disability, staying proactive about your health helps keep you on a better trajectory. What do I mean by this? Consider this graphic, which illustrates two different approaches to aging.

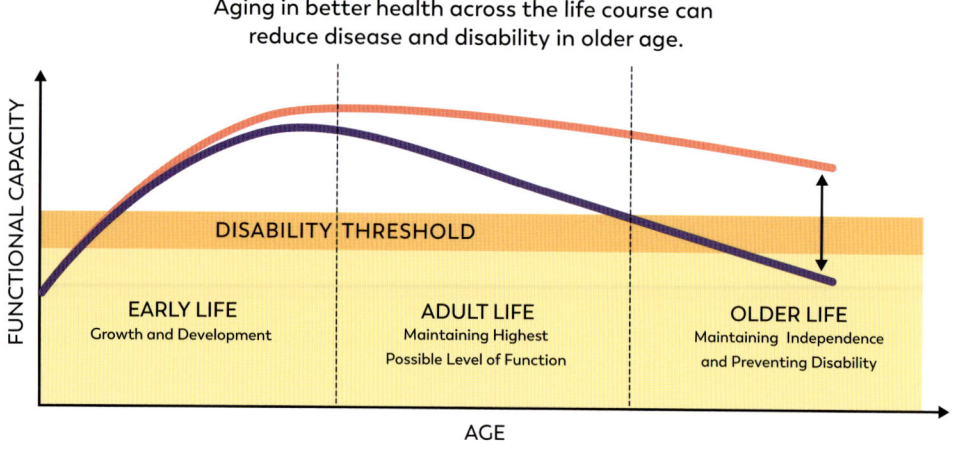

Source: Adapted from Kalache, A., Kickbush, I. A Global Strategy for Healthy Aging. *World Health*, 1997 50(4)-S.

FIGURE 3.1. Functional capacity and the aging process. Adapted from an original work published in *World Health*, a journal by the World Health Organization[1] (Creative Commons, CC BY-NC-SA 3.0 IGO).

This is a good, straightforward graphic. The two arcs represent different paths. Notice where each arc begins on the left and ends on the right.

What does a person on the top arc do well into their older age? This arc depicts an individual who prioritizes their health by staying active, being mindful of nutrition, regularly seeking professional advice, and making choices that reduce the risk of falls and injuries. While they are not perfect, they strive to maintain good habits.

What about the person on the bottom arc? There are several possibilities. This person may avoid healthy movement and dietary habits or may hesitate to seek help from health professionals. Often, they might be held back by a mental block, believing it is too late to improve their fitness. Your mental state, in terms of how you feel about exercise and sticking to good habits, is important. A mindset that dismisses the value of exercise and commitment to better health, regardless of age, can keep the person stuck in a cycle of inactivity, leading them toward the bottom arc.

Why do I say this? Internalizing negative ideas—such as "I'm not in good enough shape to work out," "I won't see results quickly enough," or "I should only do gentle movements at my age"—can create a self-fulfilling prophecy. Inactivity increases the risk of falls and injuries, makes daily tasks harder, and leads to greater physical challenges over time, eventually placing the person below the *disability threshold*. Falling below this threshold means experiencing reduced *functional capacity*—the ability to meet the physical demands of daily living without assistance.

Over time, inactivity brings a person closer to the disability threshold, which many mistakenly assume is just a part of getting older. However, it is not aging itself but rather inactivity, reinforced by negative beliefs about aging, that often contributes to disability. While it is true that our bodies change and respond differently as we age, this does not mean we should stop engaging in diverse forms of movement. On the contrary, staying active is critical for maintaining independence and enhancing quality of life.

Society often perpetuates harmful myths about aging through messages such as:

- "As we get older, things start to fall apart."
- "Falling is just part of aging."
- "Older adults should only do gentle exercises."
- "You shouldn't lift heavy weights as you age."

These ideas are simply wrong. Your life's trajectory does not have to follow the lower arc. People who stay active maintain a mindset that their best years are ahead of them and refuse to let age dictate what they are "supposed to" do or be. These rock stars choose their own adventures. While they may not all climb mountains or compete in races, they consistently engage in activities that keep their bodies fit and healthy so they can continue doing what they love—like gardening.

Gardening is a great example of how an everyday activity can keep you active and fit. Tending to a garden requires digging, bending, pulling, and lifting—all movements that build strength, balance, and flexibility. Preparing soil requires using a shovel or other tools, which demands physical strength. Planting involves bending, kneeling, or sitting on the ground, requiring flexibility and balance. Tasks like pulling weeds, watering and fertilizing plants, and harvesting also keep you moving and engaged. Gardening may not be conventional exercise, but it is an effective and rewarding way to stay active.

The level of fitness you need depends on your lifestyle. The physical demands of daily life and what constitutes being active differ from person to person, and that's okay. For some, being active might mean maintaining their home, gardening, getting around town, and attending a fitness class twice a week. For others, it might mean running marathons or hiking challenging terrain. What matters is being fit enough to meet the physical demands of daily life (what you *need* to do) as well as the physical demands of activities you love (what you *want* to do).

Staying above the disability threshold means being able to perform the activities of daily living independently. The activities you do now to stay fit and keep moving, combined with structured exercise habits, will keep you above this threshold by reducing the risk of disease and injury, so you can maintain your health, vitality, and independence. And when you can comfortably meet these daily physical demands, you are more likely to continue enjoying the activities you love—and that's the joy of movement!

Let's explore the connection between daily tasks and exercise some more. Consider carrying groceries or lifting a child. A bag of groceries or a gallon of milk weighs more than five pounds, and a child weighs much more. Each time you lift these, you are performing a version of a deadlift, row, or core exercise. Yet, many people enter a gym and limit themselves to four- or five-pound weights, believing anything heavier is "too much." But if you are already lifting heavier weights in daily life, meeting your fitness goals requires you to push beyond your comfort zone. So why not challenge yourself in the gym?

Training for the life you want means recognizing the connection between exercise and everyday activities. You want to stay strong and mobile enough to carry groceries, garden, do laundry, play with grandchildren, and much more. Adding appropriate conventional exercises to your regular routine will help you achieve this.

How fit do you need to be? To put it simply: fit enough to think less about your ability to handle life's necessities and more about other things that matter to you. Building strength and confidence takes time and effort, but the payoff is truly worthwhile.

As you set your goals, aim higher than "just fit enough." I hope you don't settle for a passing grade—strive for more!

Be Fit Enough for YOUR Life

The way you need to move your body over the course of a day is different from how someone else may need to move theirs. Each person's movement needs are unique, and it is essential to focus on practicing moving better so that you can do so with ease and confidence. The more we practice, the better prepared we are for whatever life presents us.

Sometimes, life requires us to engage in activities we don't do regularly, but we still want to be ready for those moments. For example, you may need to sprint for a short burst to catch up to someone or move quickly to avoid a collision. Below is an excerpt from an email a client sent me about an experience crossing the street.

One more example of moving easier and better happened today in downtown San Diego. I had several errands to do, and I walked from Harbor Drive up to C Street and back, crossing several intersections where I waited for the light. I noticed that when I was in the crosswalk and wanted to pick up the pace and get across faster, I really could. In the past, I could walk at whatever speed I could walk, but not faster. I had only one speed and it was slow. Today it became a game to beat the 12-second timer and then the 7-second timer, and it was so fun to see that I could do it. Besides being fun, it gave me peace of mind to know that I could move quickly if I should need to!

This client realized that she could now move quickly when needed, and that is a significant quality-of-life improvement. This is confidence—knowing that your body can respond when you need it to. Maintaining this confidence and ability can become more challenging as we age. Many older adults experience stiffness or tightness in their knees, shoulders, or hips; and chronic pain might flare up unexpectedly or in response to certain activities. Instead of getting frustrated, the best response is often to start moving more. As the saying goes: *Motion is lotion.* Moving more can be one of the best remedies for pain and stiffness, and over time it builds the confidence and motivation to tackle other things that improve your quality of life.

Start at your *good*; begin where you are. Aim to move a little more and a little better every day. Make the effort now, before an injury arises that might require physical therapy (PT). If an injury does occur and PT is prescribed, be diligent about doing your homework. I have met individuals who consistently completed their seemingly mundane PT exercises and soon fully regained their mobility and strength. I have also encountered those who found PT boring, skipped their exercises, and then wondered why their recovery didn't meet expectations. Yes, PT can be challenging, even painful, at times. Trust your qualified professional to guide you in the right direction, and don't hesitate to ask questions or seek a second opinion.

If physical therapy doesn't seem to be working as it should, despite your best efforts, don't lose hope. There are many forms of movement that people have found healing, restorative, and beneficial. Explore other options, ask questions, and most importantly, listen to your body. Be mindful of your mental and emotional states as well. Our emotions often manifest physically as tightness, pain, or fatigue. By staying aware of your body and emotions, you can find a path to healing and better movement that works for you.

Is It Too Late to Start Now?

Is it ever too late to practice better movement?

No . . . okay, next chapter.

Just kidding! It is never too late to move better. I understand how frustrating it can be when your body doesn't do what you want it to or when tasks that were once easy become challenging. However, there is also a mental game at play. If you allow a mental barrier against movement to grow—if you believe you are too old to move better—you are setting yourself on an uncomfortable path. As frustrating as it may feel, there are always opportunities to make small, incremental improvements. When taken consistently, these steps add up over time.

A great way to start is by focusing on building strength in the movements you already perform. I once had the opportunity to shadow a very accomplished trainer in the Los Angeles area who worked with clients of all ability levels, including those who were bedridden or in wheelchairs. One client, a gentleman in a wheelchair, practiced standing up, holding onto a resistance band for support, and then lowering himself as slowly as possible back into the wheelchair. This movement was challenging for him, but he worked hard at it. Over time, this simple exercise helped him strengthen his legs, arms, and core, which improved his ability to lower himself when sitting down and reduced his chances of falling. His confidence in his own abilities also increased.

Moving better and building confidence go hand in hand. Yet, confidence is often overlooked when discussing the benefits of practicing better movement. Confidence is not just a nice bonus; it is a very tangible outcome that empowers people to live life on their terms. When individuals feel confident in their ability to perform everyday tasks and engage in activities they enjoy, they are less likely to avoid movement.

One common misconception is the fear of becoming "too bulky" through strength training, which leads many people to stick to light weights and avoid challenging themselves. Let's set the record straight. You need muscle to reduce the risk or symptoms of osteoporosis, improve bone density, prevent falls, and support overall health, among other benefits. Building significant muscle bulk requires specific types of strength training, a serious time commitment at the gym, and careful attention to diet. So, put aside the fear of getting too bulky and focus instead on becoming a stronger, healthier version of yourself—before your doctor tells you that your bone density is not where it should be.

No matter your age or ability, there is always room for improvement. The key is to take small, consistent steps toward better movement and strength. The rewards—greater independence, improved health, and enhanced confidence— are well worth the effort.

Train for Adventure

Your generation is growing. Statistics show that the population of older adults in the United States is living longer than ever before.

Observe the population increase in the "Baby Boomers Turn 65" bracket in this illustration. The number of people aged sixty-five and older jumps steeply from 2010 to the projected figures for 2030—from about forty million to seventy million, a staggering increase of approximately thirty million. Now imagine an ever-expanding group of individuals succumbing to societal ideas about what they are "too old" to do. That would be a world filled with missed

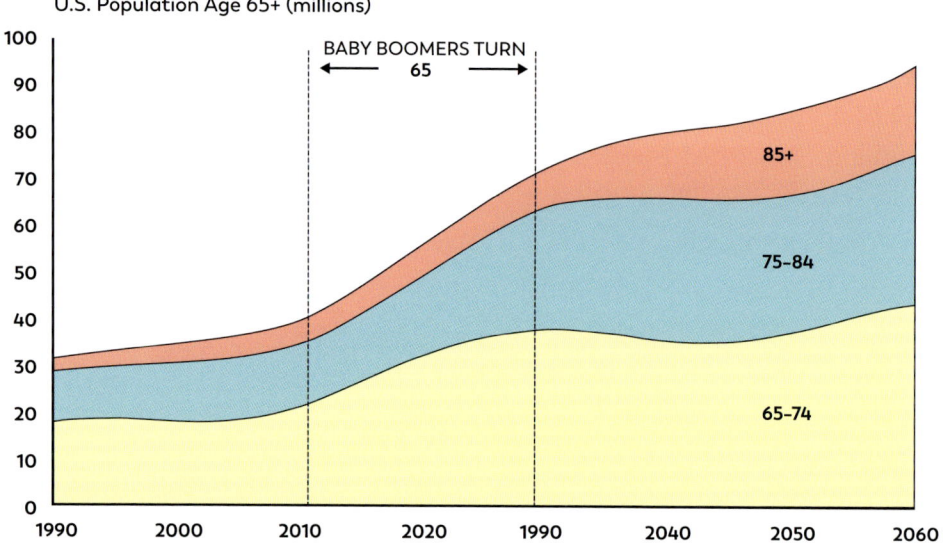

The elderly population is growing rapidly and living longer

U.S. Population Age 65+ (millions)

SOURCE: U.S. Census Bureau, National Intercensal Estimates, 2016 Population Estimates, June 2017; and National Population Projections, September 2018. Compiled by PGPF. © 2019 Peter G. Peterson Foundation

FIGURE 3.2. Estimates and projections for the population of older adults in the United States. Courtesy of Peter G. Peterson Foundation.

potential and joy. Enjoy your life. Do what you are "not supposed to do"—and train for it.

Take hiking the Grand Canyon as an example. While some might suggest sticking to a walk in the park, I say: *Why not hike the Grand Canyon?* First, focus on the logistics of your hike, including the varied and unstable terrain you will encounter on the trails. Even flat terrain can have loose gravel or dirt that may test your ability to walk confidently without falling. Hiking poles can be an excellent investment, but don't wait until the hike to use them for the first time. Practice with them beforehand to ensure they are the right height for you, which can help avoid unnecessary strain on your shoulders.

Before your trip, adjust your workouts to prepare your body for the challenge. Incorporate exercises that increase your strength and stability from head to toe. Balance exercises and drills are vital to ensure you feel steady on your feet. Depending on your chosen trail, you will need to navigate downhill slopes—and remember, you'll have to go back up too. To prepare, if you don't have hills where you live, a treadmill is a great alternative. Practice walking on it while gradually increasing and decreasing the incline to simulate walking up and downhill. Performing some variation of step-ups will also help build your single-leg strength and get you ready for uneven terrain.

Your goal is not just to get to the Grand Canyon; your goal is to *hike* it. However, the physical demands of traveling to your destination should not be overlooked. Whether you are driving or flying, travel involves walking, climbing stairs, removing shoes and jackets, and carrying bags. These movements require strength, balance, and coordination, so be sure your training includes exercises that help you handle these tasks with ease.

When you arrive, you want to fully enjoy your time at the canyon, confident in your ability to explore. Regardless of how far down the canyon you go, you will face a steady uphill climb on your way back up. I can attest that you will get caught up in the beauty as you hike down—and when you turn around and look back up at how high you started, you will revel in how far you have come and the challenge of your return journey.

Include your support team. Let your family and friends know about your plan to train for the trip. Their support and encouragement can deeply motivate you. And who knows? You might inspire them to train with you so they don't get left in the dust!

And don't forget to consult your doctor. Get the green light for any strenuous activities you are planning and seek advice for managing any issues with your knees, hips, or other problem areas. Schedule an eye exam too—clear vision is critical for navigating trails. These steps are more important than finalizing your wardrobe for the trip or stopping your mail. Focus on your body first; the other stuff can wait.

It's Never Too Late to Relearn, Unlearn, or Learn . . . If You're Open to It

You may need to relearn certain movements, like how to do a squat with less pressure on your knees. You might also need to unlearn bad habits, such as poor posture or improper techniques for lifting heavy objects. If you have used exercise machines in the past, you might need to relearn how to do a chest press with dumbbells, which requires more stabilization and coordination. You might discover that a lot more is going on in each movement than you initially realized. Take the dumbbell press, for example. It is not just about pushing the weights away from you; it also requires keeping the weights stable and aligned during the movement. You might also need to learn the proper way to breathe during exertion (hint: exhale on the effort).

You can certainly learn on your own, especially given the wealth of knowledge and advice available online. But it can feel overwhelming. Ensuring proper form can be challenging if you don't know what proper form looks like to begin with. This is where working with a trainer can help. A fitness professional can offer personalized guidance, adjust techniques or your form when necessary, and reassure you that you are on the right track. If you are feeling uncertain, seek out a trainer in your area. Trust me, we want to help you move better and with more confidence.

Invest in yourself. Learn to move with balance and strength—it's a gift that keeps on giving.

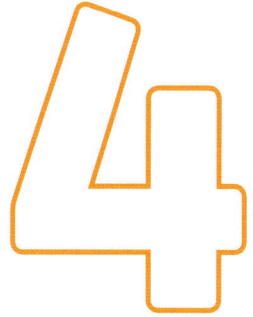

DON'T NEGLECT STRENGTH AND BALANCE TRAINING

The purpose of life is to live it.

—VIOLA DAVIS, *FINDING ME*

If you walk on the treadmill, enjoy walks with your dog, or regularly hit the trails, I applaud your consistency. But I urge you to do more. Fortify the foundation of walking by strengthening your legs through resistance training. This will ensure that you continue to walk and move better in the future.

If you have avoided strength and balance training out of fear of injury, take note: Proper training actually reduces your risk of injury. Training is not about pushing through pain. Though there may be moments of discomfort, pain and discomfort are not the same. Building strength and balance will help you move with greater ease and confidence in everyday life. When you can move your body freely and perform tasks like picking things up or climbing stairs without having to focus on the movement itself, it is easier to go about your day. Instead of worrying about physical limitations, you can focus on living. Don't wait until you reach a point where walking on inclines, stairs, or varied terrain feels impossible, limiting you to flat surfaces. Don't wait until getting out of a regular chair requires rocking yourself forward or picking up and moving simple objects becomes unmanageable. Training will help you build and maintain the abilities needed for these everyday tasks.

To be blunt, if you lack the strength and balance to perform daily activities like moving yourself and objects, someone else is likely doing these tasks for you. Independence should be your goal. While there will always be some tasks we all need help with, such as moving heavy furniture, activities like carrying groceries or retrieving canned goods from a top shelf should be within your capability.

The more we move and train our bodies, the more we will be able to do as we age. Your body is like a machine. It needs to be maintained and kept in good condition. Whether it is a sports car built for speed or a sedan that prefers the middle lane, your machine will reward you for taking care of it.

You Are Stronger Than You Think

When I work with individuals, especially during their initial sessions, we find the right weights to establish a baseline for the strength aspect of their workouts. In the gym, weights are precise—you know exactly how much they weigh. Sometimes, when I ask a client to pick a specific weight I know they are ready for, or if I pick it out for them myself, their eyes widen as they exclaim something like, "Really? [Fill-in-the-blank] pounds! That's heavy."

This hesitation is common, especially for those with a previous injury. For example, back injuries often create apprehension about lifting heavier weights. I can empathize—I have had a minor back injury myself. The fear of reinjury or making an existing issue worse is understandable. However, rebuilding confidence is key. It takes time, patience, effort, and the guidance of someone who can help you progress safely. If you avoid rebuilding your strength, you might end up moving protectively and living in a way that can ironically increase your risk of further injury. Getting stronger is a process. What matters is that you are moving in the right direction.

Some clients feel intimidated by strength training because they have not touched weights in a while. Walking, or other forms of cardio, may feel like an easier, more familiar path. So they gravitate to simpler movements that require less effort. If you identify with this, understand that strength training does not follow a rigid one-size-fits-all standard. It can be adapted to your fitness level. When working with clients new to or returning to strength training, I help them find an appropriate starting weight for each exercise. We choose a weight that challenges them without compromising their form. We stick with that weight until they can perform the exercise with ease and minimal cues from me. Progress occurs on each person's individual timeline. Once you develop better form and learn to breathe correctly while strength training, something amazing happens: You become excited about what your body can do. Confidence grows as you realize you are stronger than you initially thought.

Keep Atrophy at Bay

According to *Merriam-Webster*, atrophy is the "decrease in size or wasting away of a body part or tissue."[1] Age-related muscle mass loss is natural. But don't fall into the trap of thinking there's nothing you can do about it. Strength training is a powerful tool to counter this age-related condition. You can maintain and even improve the strength of your entire body through consistent and varied forms of strength training. Being strong enough to lift, carry, and move things—or simply to move your own body—is essential for maintaining your independence and quality of life. This is why neglecting strength training is not an option if you want to keep atrophy at bay!

For some reason, strength training is often seen as sexy, cool, and unsurprising when done by twenty- or thirty-year-olds. Yet when someone over fifty strength trains, they sometimes receive comments like "Be careful," "Do gentle exercises," or "Wow, you are strong for your age." Thankfully, attitudes are shifting. Gyms are becoming more inclusive, active older adults are becoming more visible, and the stigma around exercising as we age is diminishing. Active agers are not anomalies; they are simply doing what they should do. One of my clients, a seventy-year-old, often gets compliments about her strength and how great she looks for her age. She responds: *I don't know what seventy is supposed to look like.* Exactly. Why should being seventy mean shuffling along, doing only gentle exercises, or becoming frailer by the minute? It doesn't, and neither you nor anyone else should subscribe to that outdated idea.

Train to Move with Confidence

I want to emphasize the value of strength and balance. As you maintain and develop these through consistent and proper training, one of the most rewarding byproducts is increased confidence. I'm not just talking about feeling good or being more comfortable in your body (though those are great benefits too). I mean the confidence to move through life without hesitation. When you lack the confidence or strength to walk or climb a flight of stairs, hesitation can creep in. Along with that hesitation comes the conscious or unconscious tendency to avoid certain movements altogether or modify them in ways that feel safer, such as shuffling your feet across the floor instead of picking them up, or avoiding stairs and opting for the elevator instead.

I want you to have the confidence to move freely and without fear. However, this confidence may not come automatically, especially if you have a history of injuries or haven't moved in certain ways for a long time. It takes practice to rebuild that connection with your body. The more you practice, the more comfortable and in tune with your body you will become—and the more you will surprise yourself with what you are capable of.

Beyond Muscle: Strength Training for Bone Health

When we are younger, strength training is often focused on building stronger muscles. While this is still important as we age, training delivers another equally critical benefit: strengthening our bones. Stronger bones help lower the risk of fractures and osteoporosis. Strength training won't guarantee you will never fall, but it can mean the difference between a bruised muscle or ego and broken bones.

While nutrition also plays a role in bone health, it cannot be relied on as the sole approach for improving it. A study published in *Medicine & Science in Sports & Exercise* states that: "High-intensity resistance training, in contrast to traditional pharmacological and nutritional approaches for improving bone health in older adults, has the added benefit of influencing multiple risk factors for osteoporosis including improved strength and balance and increased muscle mass."[2] This study underscores the necessity of resistance training in building strength, balance, and muscle mass—all of which help fend off osteoporosis. If the phrase *high intensity* gives you pause, remember that intensity is subjective. What matters is using a weight that challenges while allowing you to maintain proper form. I understand that some people feel hesitant about resistance training because they have previously injured themselves while working out at the gym or exercising alone. If this is you, consider working with a fitness professional to build your confidence. Start by finding your baseline— the weight that challenges you without compromising your form. Track your progress and understand that moving to heavier weights is something you must *earn* through consistent practice and mastery of form. Attempting to lift too much too soon can lead to compensations in your movements and form, potentially leading to injury later. Let's also dispel the myth of "no pain, no gain." A solid, challenging workout does not need to leave you limping out the door. Progress should come from consistent effort, not unnecessary strain.

Strength Train for Independence

You want to do what you want to do on your terms. Asking for help with tasks you have always done—like getting out of a chair or lifting something from the floor to a counter—can be a sign that your physical limitations, such as a lack of strength, are impacting your autonomy. A study published in *Gerontology* captured this perfectly: "Low strength is a primary limiting factor for functional independence."[3]

While this study touched on many other aspects of movement, such as neuromotor functions, gait, and aerobic fitness, it emphasized how developing lower extremity muscle groups through strength training can contribute to preventing functional decline. Why is lower-body strength so important? Because many essential movements—walking, squatting, climbing stairs, stepping to the side, and hinging the hips back to pick something up— depend on the strength of the hips and legs. If these movements become difficult or impossible, it may signal the onset of functional decline. By prioritizing strength training, particularly for the lower body, you can maintain or even regain your ability to perform these everyday activities, preserving your independence.

Strength Train for Heart Health

It is a common misconception that cardio and strength training are entirely separate forms of exercise—running versus lifting weights. Many people believe you cannot gain cardiovascular benefits from strength training. That is simply not true. Strength training can get your heart rate up and provide a cardiovascular workout. In their book *The Barbell Prescription*, Jonathon M. Sullivan and Andy Baker delve into this fallacy directly: "For a long time, the conventional wisdom held that, while resistance training could certainly make for stronger muscles and bones, it didn't train the heart or promote cardiovascular health."[4] If you have thought this way, you are not alone. Many share this false belief. However, those who have participated in circuit-based group classes like CrossFit or Orangetheory Fitness likely know firsthand that strength training can elevate your heart rate. These classes combine strength training and cardio or feature strength training exercises performed under timed conditions or for repetitions, with timed rest. Of course, you can practice such a workout on your own outside of a group class and achieve similar results, including the cardiovascular benefit.

Sullivan and Baker also discuss how research is changing the outdated view of strength training's cardiovascular benefits by studying the relationship between resistance training and cardiovascular fitness. One study cited in the book highlights that "both endurance training and strength training produced similar structural cardiac adaptations."[5] This means that strength training is not only good for your muscles and bones but also benefits your heart. Don't fall into the trap of loading up on conventional cardio and neglecting strength training. You might be surprised at how taxing a set of squats or chest presses can be, especially when performed with proper intensity and form.

You need cardiorespiratory training in your life for heart health. Activities such as brisk walking, stationary bike intervals, or jogging are excellent choices. However, it is equally important to supplement your cardio with strength training. One key point I want to emphasize is *intensity*. If you are doing conventional cardio at a pace that allows you to hold a conversation without effort, you are likely not pushing hard enough. Similarly, if you are lifting weights that don't challenge you while maintaining proper form, the weights are not heavy enough. Whatever exercise you choose, challenge yourself. Push your limits safely and effectively to gain the full benefit of your workout.

The Stability Connection

Let's define stability. At its core, stability is the ability to *own* a position—to maintain control and balance while holding or transitioning through a position. Here are some real-life examples:

- Picking up luggage, lifting it above your head, and sliding it into an overhead bin.

- Picking up and holding out a baby to hand over to a friend or family member.

Stability is not just about moving something or yourself. It is also about having the control to move slowly or with precision, hold a position, or carry an object without risking injury or compensating.

Some machine-based exercises can help you improve stability. But I challenge you to step away from machines to enhance your stability even further. For instance, the seated chest press machine can strengthen your shoulders, chest, and other muscles involved in pushing. However, when you translate that movement to pressing two dumbbells on an inclined bench, you add a new layer of challenge. You are not just pressing weights; you are also working on your grip and controlling the movement to keep the dumbbells aligned. This requires you to be careful not to let the dumbbells tilt or cave inward toward your thumbs and down to your chest, or out toward your pinkies and away from your chest. This type of training improves your stability and ability to own the position without compensation or injury.

Balance: The Critical Program Running in the Background

Just as your computer and phone run many programs in the background—which you might notice only when they slow down your device—your body also has a program that operates in the background: balance.

Think about your typical day. You head out to run a shopping errand. You walk to your car, shift items in your hands, open your car door, and get in. You drive to the store, shop for what you need, and return home. Through all these actions, the "balance program" works in the background to keep you steady—adjusting for every step, weight shift, and carried object.

We typically notice our balance only when it becomes the focus of a movement or if it becomes a concern. For instance, you might notice it when walking on a narrow surface, balancing on one foot, or catching yourself from a potential fall. If your ability to maintain balance while moving has eroded, everyday tasks like changing direction quickly, getting in and out of a chair, or even walking briskly can feel unstable, indicating the need for balance training.

Neglecting balance training will eventually increase your risk of falls. Don't wait until you notice your balance isn't what it used to be. Start challenging and improving it today, regardless of your current ability. Fancy equipment isn't necessary. Here are two simple exercises to get you started:

- **Tightrope walk.** Imagine walking a tightrope. Keep your hands by your sides, relax, and walk forward heel to toe slowly, because speed hides control. Then try walking backward in the same manner.

- **Side step with glute engagement.** Stand in neutral position with your feet close together. Step out to the side with your right foot. Sink your hips back to engage your glutes. Push off with your right foot to come back up to the starting position.

You will find that balance is a recurring theme throughout this book because it is fundamental to better movement. Being strong is excellent, and being able to press 200 lbs. on a leg press is impressive. But can you walk upstairs without holding on to the railing? Balance is often overlooked in workouts. Lifting weights, going for a run, or playing sports often take precedence when our balance is pretty good; so we take it for granted.

Regardless of where you stand on the strength or balance spectrum, find a way to strength train that also improves your balance. There are always ways to modify movements (I call them *options*) to safely challenge yourself while enhancing how you balance and move.

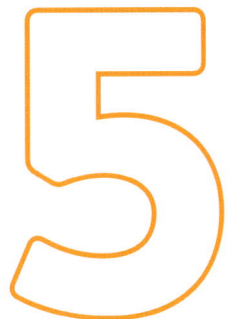

THERE ARE ALWAYS OPTIONS TO A MOVEMENT

> *I take great issue with the term "anti-aging." The way I see it, you have two choices in life: You can either get older, or die.*
>
> —HELEN MIRREN, INTERVIEW BY BRIAN UNDERWOOD, *OPRAH DAILY*

Think of improving your movement and exercise as a choose-your-own-adventure opportunity. There are always ways to make something easier or more difficult. When working on your mobility, it is important not to feel restricted by a video you watched or what you saw someone doing at the gym. A common phrase in the fitness industry (and likely in other fields too) is to "meet someone where they are." For trainers, this means presenting exercises that match the client's current physical abilities.

If you are reading this book to learn how to exercise on your own, you are essentially your own trainer. Begin your exercise journey at your *good*—your baseline. But how do you figure out your baseline? Let's use squats as an example. Can you perform twelve squats to the depth of an average chair? If not, that is a great starting point. Find a chair without wheels, place its back against a wall, and take a seat. Then, stand up and sit back down, repeating this twelve times. Make sure you don't rock to stand up or plop into the chair when descending to sit. If this seated version is manageable, that is your baseline. If squats without a chair feel easy, try holding a weight in your hands. A good baseline means exerting effort, but the first attempt should not feel exhausting. By the last repetition, however, it should feel challenging.

Let's consider a practical example. Imagine you are a trainer working with a client named Mary, who is seventy-five years old. She believes she cannot do squats because they are harmful to her due to arthritis in one of her knees. Although she is retired, Mary remains active and enjoys helping at her neighborhood garden. Here is a multiple-choice question about her first session: What exercise would you choose for Mary?

A. No squats for Mary—keep her seated for all her exercises because she's too old.

B. Make her do squats holding a 20 lb. dumbbell, just like you do.

C. Have her perform squats using a properly sized chair, standing up from the chair and sitting back down.

D. Avoid squats altogether because they are bad for Mary's knees.

The best answer is option C. This option builds Mary's confidence in her ability to perform squats. Performing squats without a chair might make her uncomfortable due to her knee condition. Also, since she is active and enjoys gardening, this exercise supports her ability to continue those activities. Now, why are the other answers not ideal?

- **Option A.** This option is ageist and dismissive. You may have ruled out this option as soon as you read it. Believe it or not, many people mistakenly believe this.

- **Option B.** This answer is unrealistic. Don't expect your clients—or yourself—to work out like someone else. Meet them where they are. And, likewise, start at your *good*.

- **Option D.** This option is misguided. It reinforces Mary's incorrect belief that squats are bad for her. She already performs similar movements daily, such as sitting or standing from a chair and using the bathroom. Helping her understand this could motivate her.

There are several ways for Mary to perform squats. She could hold onto something, like a strong resistance band secured to a sturdy pole, which would help her stand up and sit down more comfortably by taking some pressure off her knees. She could also use a firm cushion on the chair to reduce seat depth, making the descent and ascent easier. Over time, as her strength improves, the cushion can be removed or replaced with a thinner one, increasing the challenge.

We want to avoid letting Mary rock to get out of the chair, which indicates a lack of leg strength or balance. Speed can hide control. When we rely on speed or momentum to perform movements, we often sacrifice control, leading to accidents. Our goal for Mary is to enable her to stand up from a chair, pick things off the ground, and move during daily activities with control. That said, there are situations where power and speed are beneficial—like when opening a stuck fridge door or raking leaves. However, for movements with precision, such as gently placing a toddler down, control is crucial.

If the concept of adapting exercises does not resonate, consider this: How many ways can you make eggs? Scrambled, fried, boiled—the options are endless, and each person has their preference. Some methods of cooking eggs may require specialty equipment, while others only need an average skillet or pot. The same applies to fitness. There are countless ways to perform exercises and many great tools to help you move better. The goal is to find what works best for you with the resources you have. If you don't have the right tools, adapt and adjust. If you don't have the answers, ask those who do.

Certain movements can enhance our ability to perform an exercise, such as the squat. Consider these three images of Anthony sitting on a chair, positioned in a free-standing high squat without a chair, and lastly, positioned with his hands and knees on the floor.

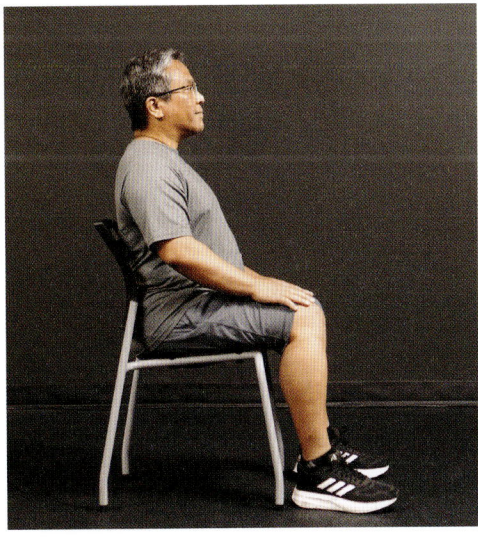
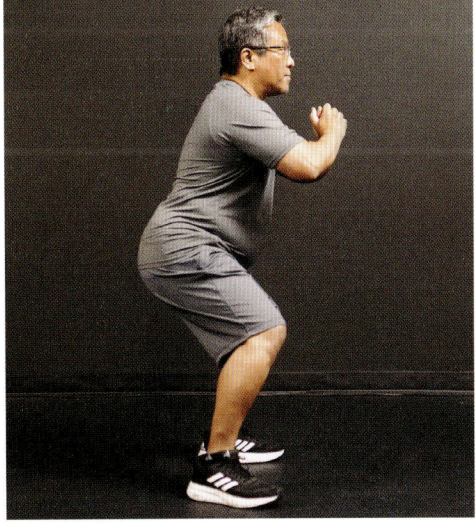

FIGURE 5.1.   **FIGURE 5.2.**

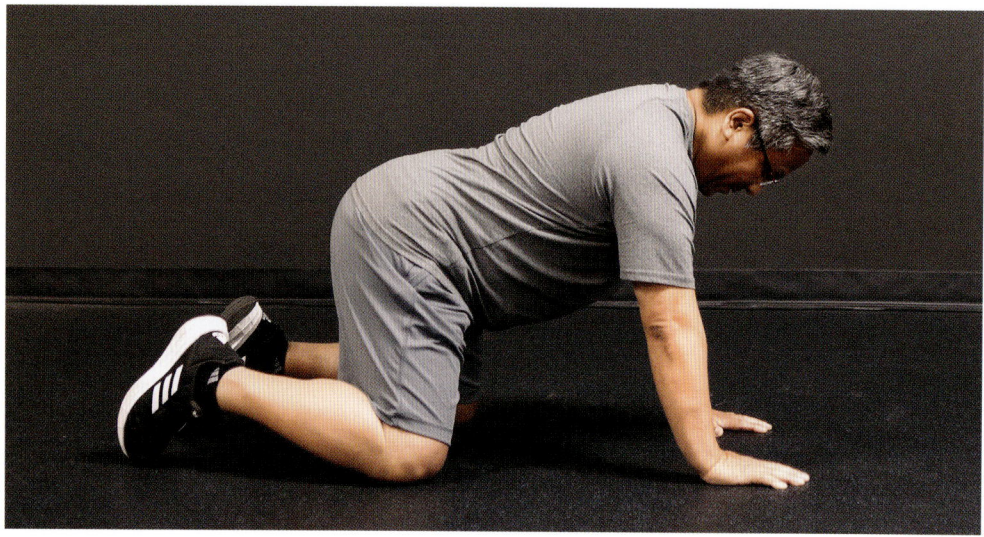

FIGURE 5.3.

These movements differ, yet they share some similarities. Pay attention to the position of the lower half of his body. When he is on his hands and knees, he does not encounter the downward force experienced in a free-standing squat. However, rocking back and forth on all fours can help lubricate the joints involved in squatting, which in turn can improve flexibility, enhance squat performance, and prepare the body for more challenging movements. If putting pressure on your knees is uncomfortable, try placing a towel under them or performing the exercise on a carpet or rug.

You may wonder how the squats with and without a chair are alike. The primary difference is that the chair provides a predetermined depth and support during practice. When clients follow the cues not to rock back to stand up or plop down into the chair, they avoid using momentum or gravity to perform the movement. Both variations allow for practicing proper form, as each requires hinging the hips back to go lower, before standing back up.

Practicing different options for a movement can help you overcome the "I used to be able to do that, but I can't now" mentality. Permit yourself to move according to your current physical abilities. Once you set that foundation, you can gradually progress to more challenging variations without compromising your form.

Let's revisit our training scenario with Mary. Starting her practice with squats using a chair and cushion is a suitable first step. She may initially struggle, which is part of the learning process, but this adjusted option is attainable for her. As her posture and form improve, the next step could be to remove the cushion or replace it with a thinner one, increasing the challenge by lowering the depth of her squat. This gradual progression will require her to use her leg strength more, further building both her strength and confidence. The journey to better movement is about consistent, incremental progress. Small steps lead to big improvements over time.

Strength Training and Options

When we think of strength training, we often picture machines, barbells, or dumbbells. These can be effective tools for building strength, but there are great alternatives as well. Resistance bands, for instance, are a fantastic option. They come in various levels of resistance, with heavier bands providing more resistance. Additionally, resistance bands are portable, making them ideal for travel when access to a gym is limited. Another great alternative is Total Body Resistance Exercise, commonly known as TRX. Many gyms offer TRX suspension training systems, and you can request a private session to learn how to use them effectively. If you prefer to learn on your own, YouTube videos or phone-based fitness applications can provide helpful coaching. TRX and other suspension-based exercise systems have an easy learning curve and offer user-friendly ways to increase strength and flexibility for people of all ages and fitness levels. These systems also travel well since they can be anchored to ceilings, doors, strong beams, or even trees, providing versatility.

Here are a few examples of strength training that don't require machines or dumbbells:

- Resistance tubing (resistance bands with handles)
- Strength or resistance bands (large rubber bands without handles)
- Bodyweight exercises (using your own weight for resistance)
- TRX (a suspension-based training system)
- Slam balls (weighted balls designed not to bounce)
- Medicine balls (weighted balls that bounce)
- Sandbags (versatile weights for various movements)

Balance Training and Options

I cannot overemphasize the importance of balance for movement and stability. Balance training is essential for navigating daily life with confidence, regardless of age or fitness level. I encourage everyone to regularly challenge and train their balance. As someone who runs half-marathons every year, I can attest that the better my balance, the smoother my running performance. When running, only one foot is on the ground at any given time, making balance crucial for ensuring smooth, efficient movement. I encourage runners to engage in exercises that test their balance to reinforce their confidence.

Here are some options to work on balance, beyond simply standing on one leg:

- **Half-kneeling.** Use a yoga mat or towel under your knee. Ensure both legs form right angles, with your hips, knees, and feet aligned. Maintain a tall posture and steady breathing. Surprisingly, holding this position can be more challenging than it seems.

- **Staggered stance.** From a standing position, bring one foot about two feet behind you. Lock your back knee and balance on the ball of your back foot. Keep your front foot firmly flat on the ground with the knee slightly bent but not locked above your ankle. Stay tall and breathe steadily.

- **Lateral step to balance.** From standing, step to the side as far as is comfortable. Push off with your moving foot and raise it to balance on the other foot. If needed, perform the movement in steps and keep your hands on a stable surface, like a countertop, for support in case you lose your balance.

You can find demonstrations of these exercises and more in the "Instructional Videos" section on my website, www.incrementalfit.com.

While static balance exercises, like standing on one leg, are a good starting point, they are just the tip of the iceberg when it comes to challenging and improving your balance. Balance is used even more when we are in motion, so I like to introduce some controlled movements during balance training when I work with clients to greatly enhance its benefits. You really don't have to stand on a raised surface to do balance training. My clients can attest that balance training can be adequately challenging and incredibly effective on a flat surface. One client found walking in tandem (heel to toe) and standing on one leg to be difficult, yet his previous trainer had him using a Bosu ball (a raised curved half-dome) for balance training. While such tools can be helpful, they are not necessary—and in some situations, they may not be appropriate. In his case, the floor provided more than enough of a challenge, and using a raised curved surface was not suitable yet. The goal is steady improvement, not unnecessary risks.

Cardio and Options

Cardiovascular training, or cardio, has its place in fitness and offers many great benefits, especially for heart health. Some of you are likely looking for guidance on incorporating it effectively into your exercise routine. However, in my experience, women often overdo cardio while neglecting strength training, whereas men tend to skip cardio entirely and focus solely on strength workouts. A balanced approach is key—meeting in the middle ensures you are not neglecting either aspect of fitness. If you are training for races or other endurance events, cardio will naturally be a significant part of your regimen, but strength training should never be overlooked!

Here are some tips and options for effective cardio:

- **Variation is your friend.** Avoid falling into a monotonous routine of walking on a treadmill or running outside aimlessly. Time your sessions and track your distance covered. Add shorter, faster-paced runs or walks. Incorporate inclines to make your routine more challenging.

- **Take it outside.** Go for a brisk walk. You should barely be able to hold a conversation. Ditch your phone to maintain focus and fully enjoy the experience.

- **Dance classes.** Have fun while getting your heart rate up.

- **Join a sports league.** Participating in activities like tennis is excellent for building endurance and provides a social element.

- **Hiking.** Enjoy nature while challenging yourself on various terrains.

- **Exercise machines.** Bikes, ellipticals, and rowers are great for cardio, but make sure you maintain proper form to prevent injuries.

Stretching and Options

We all need to stretch. It is often overlooked, but I believe it is as vital as staying hydrated. Just as drinking water one day doesn't carry over to the next, stretching requires our ongoing attention. If you are diligent about working out but don't stretch or work on mobility, this inattentiveness can add up over time—a nail in a tire may not cause a flat right away, but it will eventually.

Tight muscles or fascia restrict our range of motion and increase the risk of injury. Over the years, we may even get accustomed to this reduced range of motion, thinking it's normal. However, it can negatively impact our posture and movement during daily activities like driving, sitting, talking on the phone, walking, etc. Regular stretching helps reset your body and breath, increases blood flow, and facilitates optimal muscle and joint function.

So, how should you stretch? There isn't a single way to stretch; many options are available including yoga or Pilates classes, using equipment like foam rollers, or bodyweight stretches without any equipment. If you have back pain or injuries, seek professional guidance to ensure your stretches are safe and effective.

People often forget to breathe while stretching. When experiencing pain or trying new movements, we tend to focus so intently that we hold our breath. Learning to breathe better can significantly enhance your stretches. If you practice yoga or similar modalities, you understand that breathing is an integral part of the stretch. The technique of "breathing into the stretch" helps you relax and settle deeper into the stretch. Try holding your breath during a stretch, and then compare that to gently inhaling and exhaling as you stretch—it can be a game changer.

Regular stretching fosters staying in touch with your body as well as body awareness. As you focus on stretching different sides and at different angles, you may notice tight areas or imbalances between your limbs or sides of your body. The more you improve body awareness, the greater your insight into the connections between your workouts, stretches, and overall movements during the rest of the day, which can further guide your workouts and everyday movements.

A note for hyperflexible folks and stretching enthusiasts: You are likely familiar with the benefits of stretching and enjoy doing it frequently. But please don't overdo it. Take a day off from stretching occasionally and balance it with strength training. Think of your body as a tree that can bend flexibly in the wind. You can only bend so far without breaking; you need to be strong enough to remain stable and in control.

There Are Always Options

If you have joint issues or injuries, such as sore knees, hips, or shoulders, your exercise options may feel limited. However, there is always a way to adapt and learn a new or better way to move. This could mean relearning proper form or learning stretching and mobility drills to increase range of motion and reduce pain. Consistent practice is key to seeing results. The more regularly you practice, the better you will feel and move in everyday life. Results take time, but every small effort adds up. Give yourself permission to learn, make mistakes, and improve. Instead of viewing modifications as an easier way or "not the real way" of doing an exercise, think of them as variations that meet you where you are in your fitness journey.

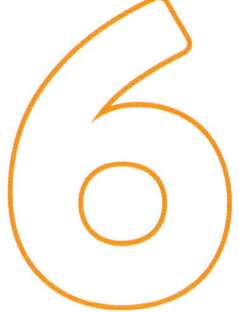

PHOTO INTERMISSION

As the popular adage goes, a picture is worth a thousand words. This chapter introduces visuals that illustrate movements we commonly encounter in everyday life outside the gym. Alongside these images, I discuss the exercises that often go unnoticed but correspond to these real-life actions. This connection emphasizes the power and importance of exercise for older adults. By practicing and improving these movements through the exercises explained here, you can enhance your ability to perform daily tasks safely and efficiently.

Keep this straightforward diagram in mind as you view the photos in this chapter. It shows how exercise and real-life movements overlap. Of course, this intersection will differ for everyone. In a gym or exercise setting, we practice form, breathing, and technique in a controlled environment. In contrast, real-life situations involve other objects and terrains. Yet, the more we practice optimal movement patterns during exercise, the better they carry over to our daily lives.

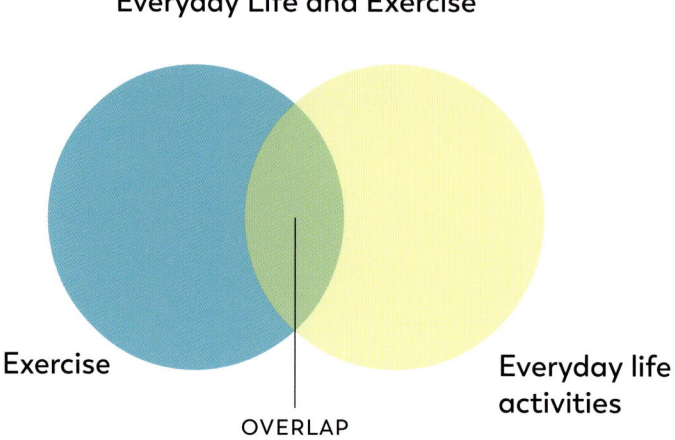

FIGURE 6.1.

REAL-LIFE SCENARIO: CHECKING THE AIR IN YOUR CAR TIRE

This is a common task for car owners. Whether you are checking the tire pressure or inspecting something underneath your car, this action involves movements that resemble specific exercises.

What I See: One movement mirrors a squat, while the other resembles a half-kneeling to standing movement.

- **Squat.** The squat is a fundamental movement used daily. It involves lowering ourselves to a seated position and then standing back up. The depth of the squat can vary, such as sitting on a low chair or higher, as shown in the image. This everyday movement occurs when we descend onto a chair or the floor, get back up, or use the toilet. Sometimes, we lower and raise ourselves with assistance, like holding onto something for support. Other times, we must manage without assistance, which requires greater strength and balance.

- **Half-kneeling to standing.** This movement involves balance and what fitness professionals call a *progression*. Progression simply means making an exercise more challenging as your abilities improve. While standing and balancing on one leg may be easy for some, transitioning from a half-kneeling position to standing adds an extra challenge that strengthens your foundation. Practicing this progression ensures you can return to a standing position confidently with fewer balance issues, reducing your risk for falls.

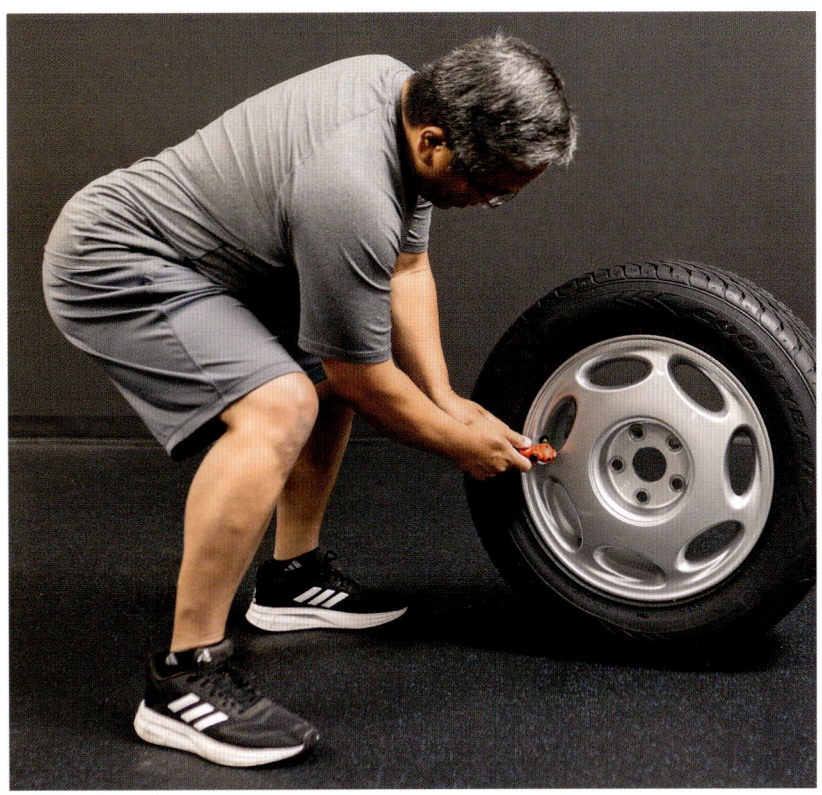

FIGURE 6.2.

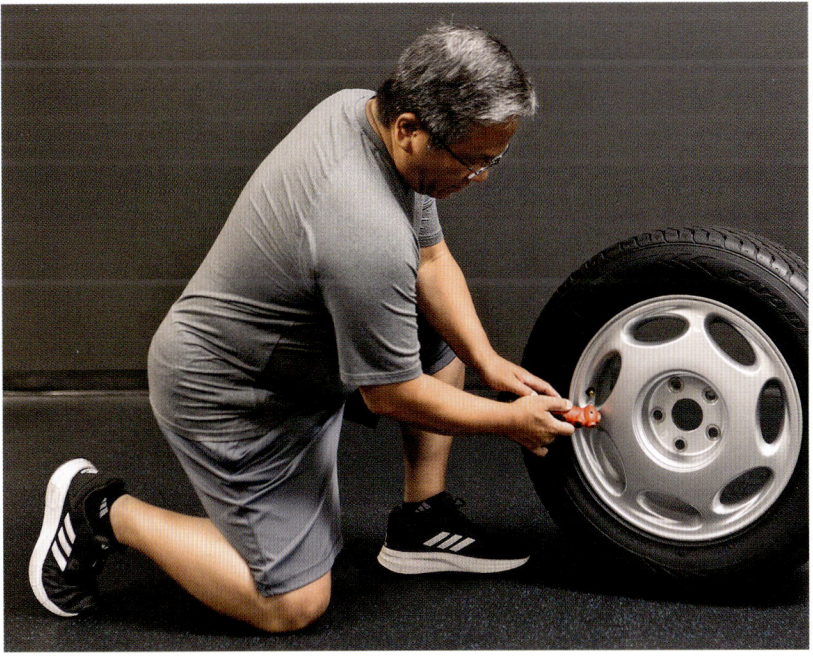

FIGURE 6.3.

Let's take a closer look at the *half-kneeling movement.* In the following sequence, Anthony is holding a ten-pound medicine ball. Holding a weight during certain exercises provides several benefits: It engages the core, especially when holding the weight away from your body. It helps us maintain better posture during the movement without needing reminders to do so. It is good practice for real-world situations where we often move while carrying objects in our hands.

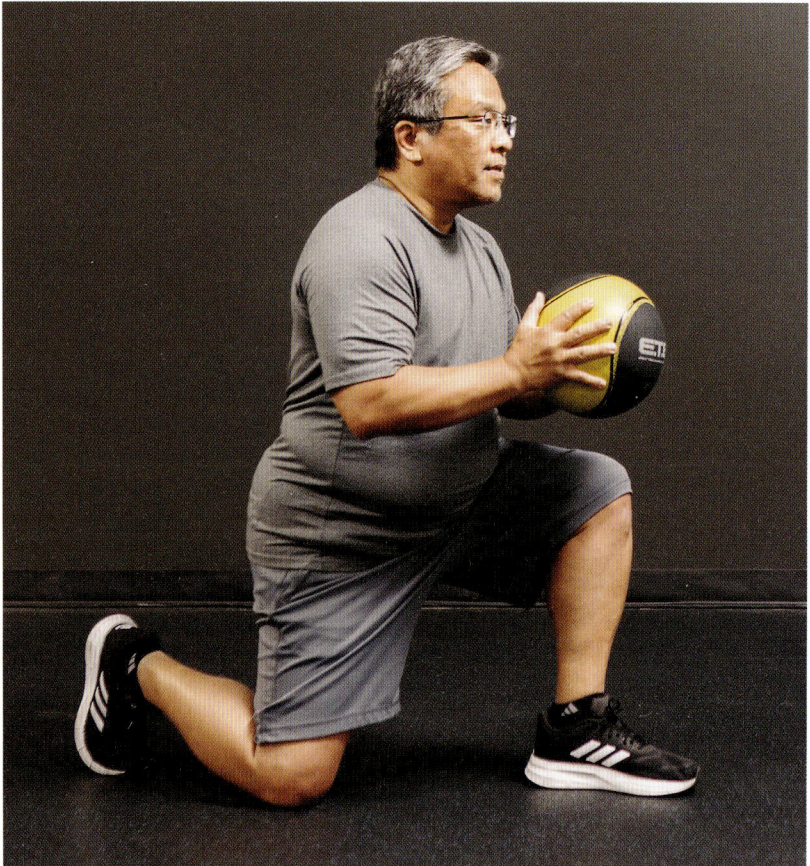

FIGURE 6.4.

Here, Anthony is in a half-kneeling position, similar to when he is checking the air pressure in the tire. Notice his tall posture and the alignment of his upper body. When performing tasks like checking tire pressure, you typically lean forward and turn toward the tire. However, when preparing to stand up from this position, starting with a tall posture is optimal for better control and alignment.

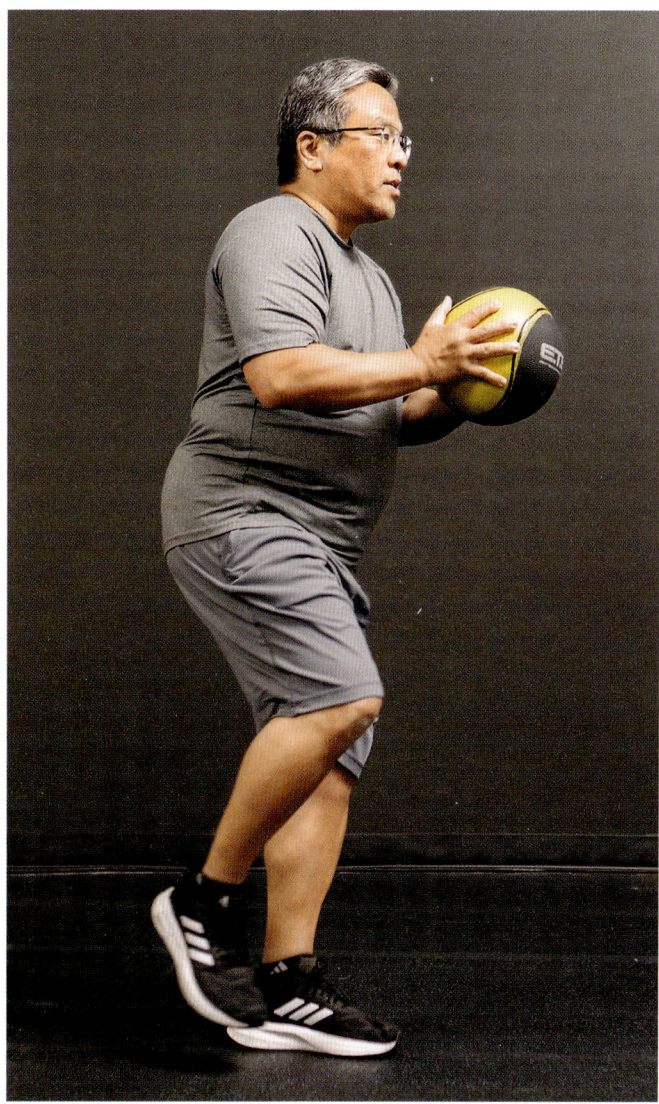

FIGURE 6.5.

This is an action shot of Anthony in the process of standing up from the half-kneeling position. He is mid-motion, balancing on one foot with his other foot lifted off the ground. He has not yet reached a fully upright, tall position. In real-life scenarios, such as standing after checking your tires, you typically wouldn't pause while balancing at the end, yet balance is called on. Pausing mid-motion while balancing before fully standing increases the difficulty of the movement. As I always say, make your exercises challenging so that real-life movements are not.

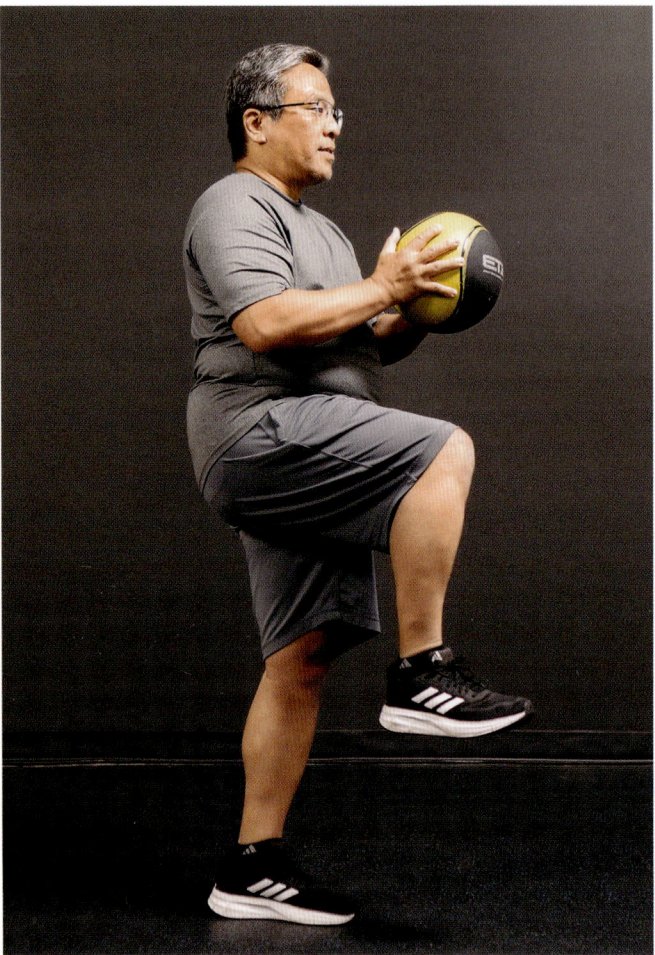

FIGURE 6.6.

Now, Anthony has reached the final standing and balancing position. He remains tall while balancing on one leg, with his opposite knee raised to hip level. I don't expect you to perform this exercise with spot-on form right away; the goal is to work toward achieving it.

REAL-LIFE SCENARIO: LIFTING A BABY (OR A TEN-POUND BAG OF SOIL)

Sometimes, life requires us to lift something delicate—whether it is a baby, a bag of soil, a pet, or any fragile item that needs careful handling to avoid damage or spills. The key is not just to lift but to carry and move with care and control, ensuring the item (or baby!) stays secure and undisturbed.

Here's how this plays out . . .

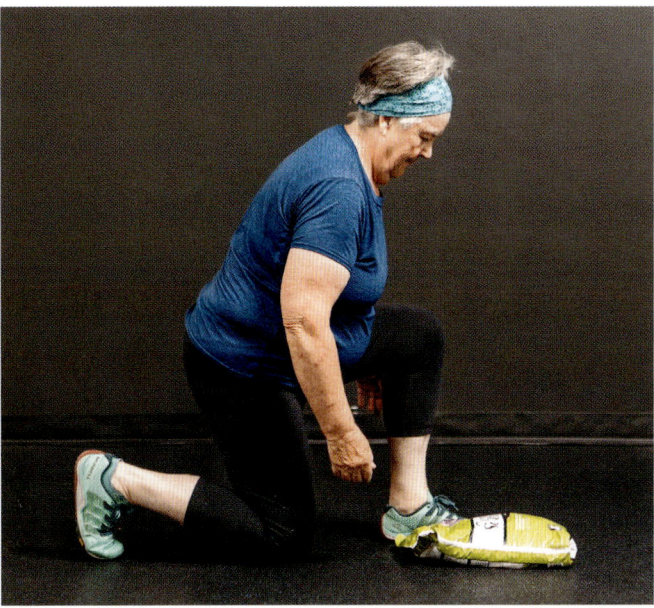

FIGURE 6.7.

At the start, Martha assumes a half-kneeling position, preparing to lift the bag. This position ensures stability and allows her to use her legs and hips effectively, rather than overloading her back.

As she picks up the bag, notice how she cradles it securely against her forearm. This technique reduces strain on her arms and shoulders while keeping the item stable.

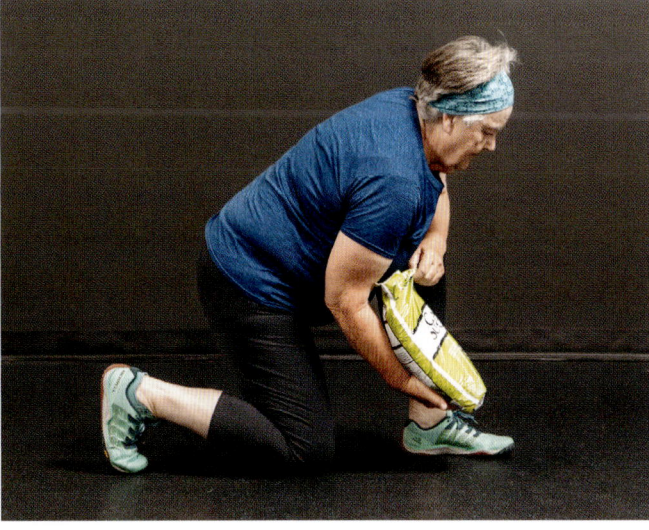

FIGURE 6.8.

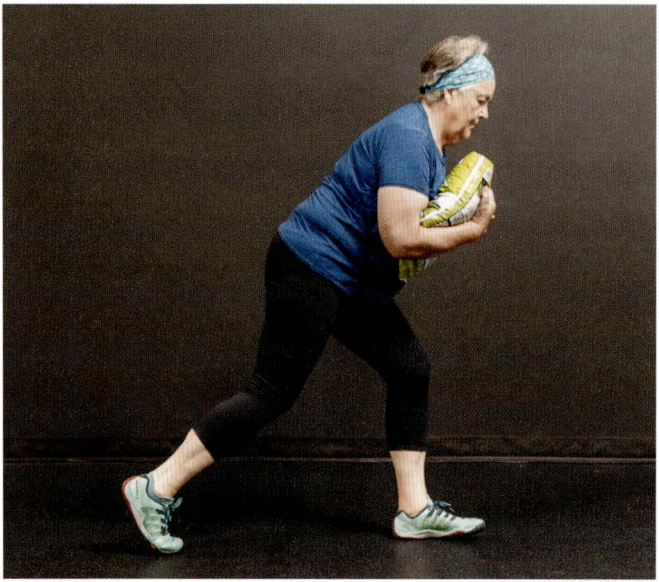

FIGURE 6.9.

Here, she is in the process of standing up from the half-kneeling position. She uses her legs to drive upward while maintaining control of the bag, focusing on moving deliberately and securely.

Now fully upright, she is in a stable position, holding the bag securely. From here, Martha would place the bag (or baby) back down with care, ensuring control at every step.

What I See: At its core, this is a floor-to-standing movement, but with added complexity due to the fragile item being held. Controlled movement is critical in this process. Now, let's explore how I train clients to prepare for floor-to-standing movements using an exercise called the *Turkish get-up*. Don't be intimidated by how complex it may seem; it simply involves getting up from the ground to standing while holding a weight (or object). This exercise

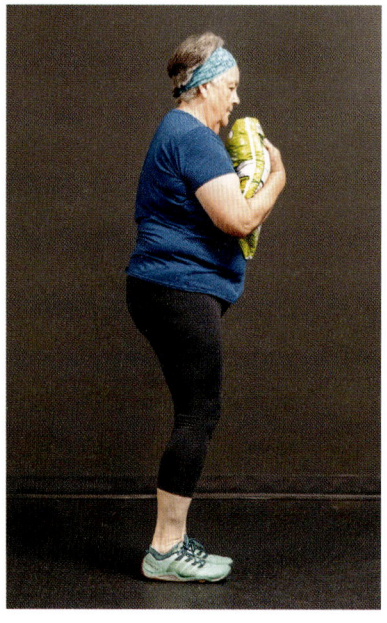

FIGURE 6.10.

challenges the entire body and promotes strength, balance, and coordination. As with the previously discussed exercise, this should also be practiced in a way that challenges you more than moving in everyday life. Not everyone needs to perform the full Turkish get-up. For clients with significant joint issues or conditions like vertigo, I modify or simplify the movements. Regardless of their abilities, all my clients practice floor-to-standing transitions in some form during our sessions. I am just sneaky that way.

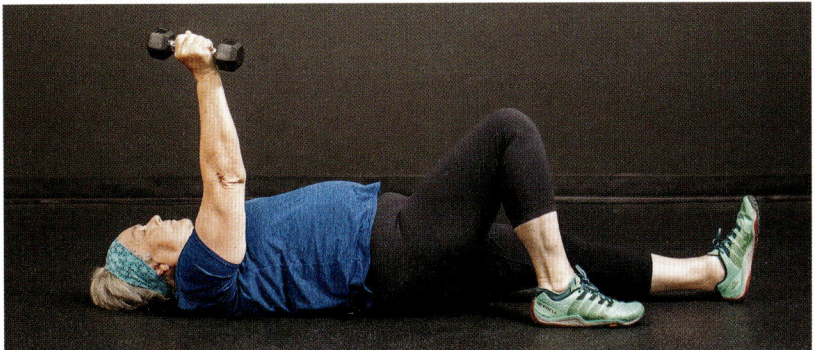

FIGURE 6.11.

Martha is working hard from the start, even while lying on her back. The raised 5 lb. dumbbell challenges her shoulder and core to maintain stability. This weight is suitable for Martha and reminds her just enough that it is there.

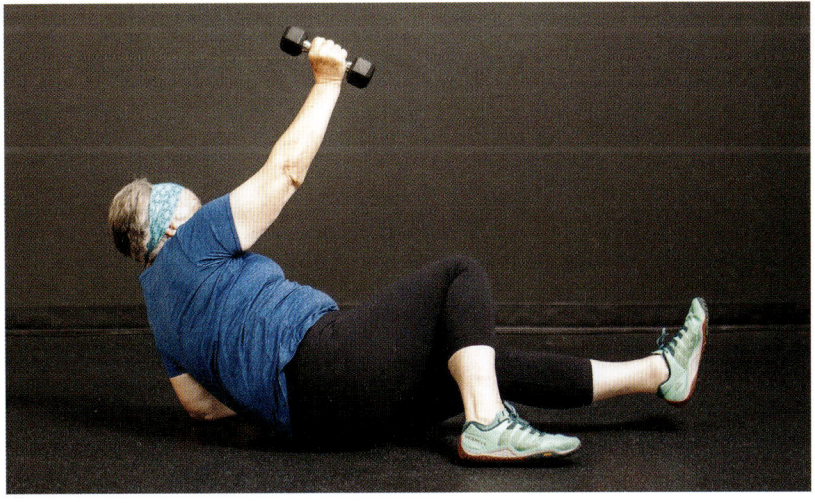

FIGURE 6.12.

In this step, the core and both shoulders are fully engaged. The right arm remains raised throughout the exercise. Notice how her left forearm and hand are planted on the ground, with the left elbow locked and the left shoulder engaged. Her right foot is flat on the ground, and the right leg, hip, and glute are also actively working to provide stability and support for the next transition.

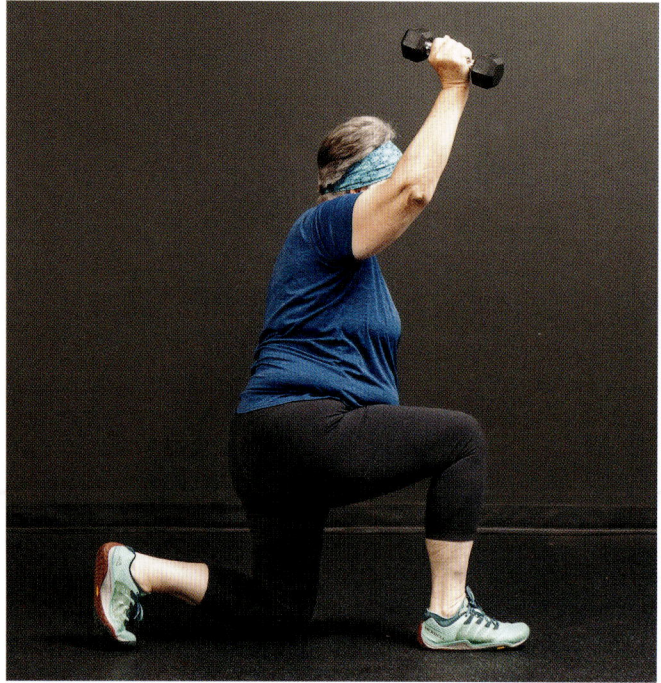

FIGURE 6.13.

Boom! Martha is now in the half-kneeling position. To get to this position, she pushed off her right foot and lifted her hips, giving her left foot adequate clearance to go under and move into a flexed position on the ground. Her left hand remained on the ground for support until she reached this tall, upright stance. At this point, she is working on balance, and one side of her core (known as the obliques) is really fired up to keep her torso tall and her shoulders square while stabilizing the dumbbell above her head.

This movement, minus the overhead weight, mirrors the initial steps involved in picking up the bag of soil. Having established the connection between the Turkish get-up and picking up objects off the floor, I like to think of the actions leading up to this step as extra credit.

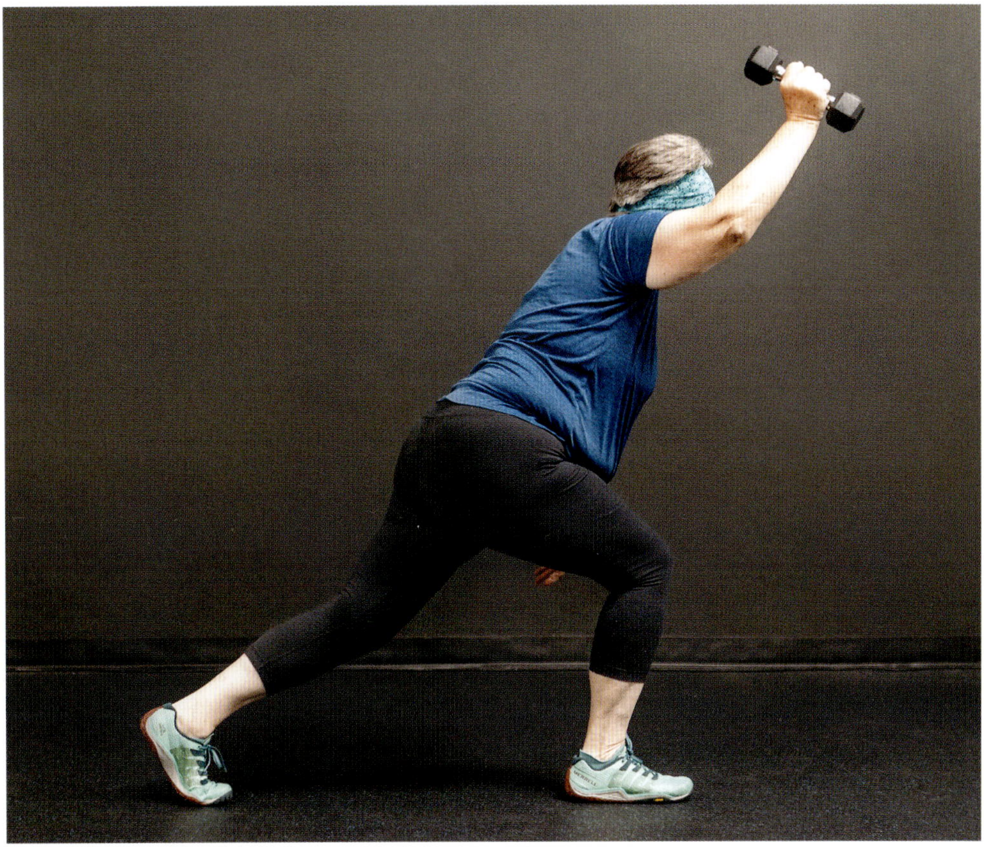

FIGURE 6.14.

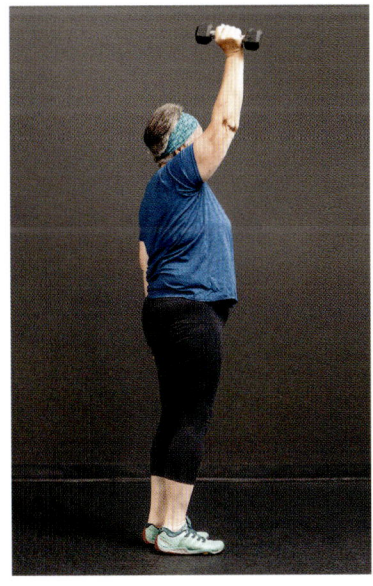

FIGURE 6.15.

This action shot captures Martha transitioning from half-kneeling to standing. Her left knee is now off the ground, with only her left toes and right foot in contact with the ground. Her right leg and hip, as well as her left foot, drive the movement and provide stability, while her left leg engages to stabilize and maintain balance. She continues to support the weight overhead, further challenging her shoulder and core muscles.

Standing tall, Martha maintains a strong posture. Her right shoulder is still engaged to sustain stability while she holds the dumbbell.

Now, she will return to the ground in reverse order. This half of the exercise also requires stability, strength, balance, and coordination, just like during the get-up phase. The controlled descent mirrors placing the bag of soil back on the ground up to the half-kneeling position but adds movements beyond that.

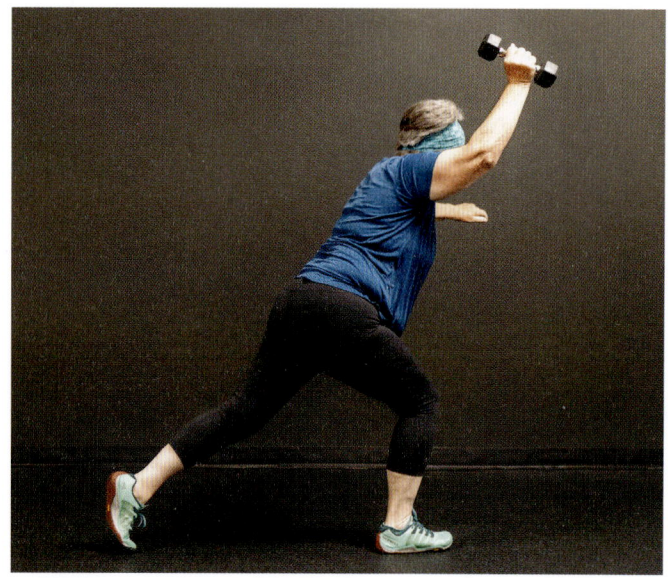

FIGURE 6.16.

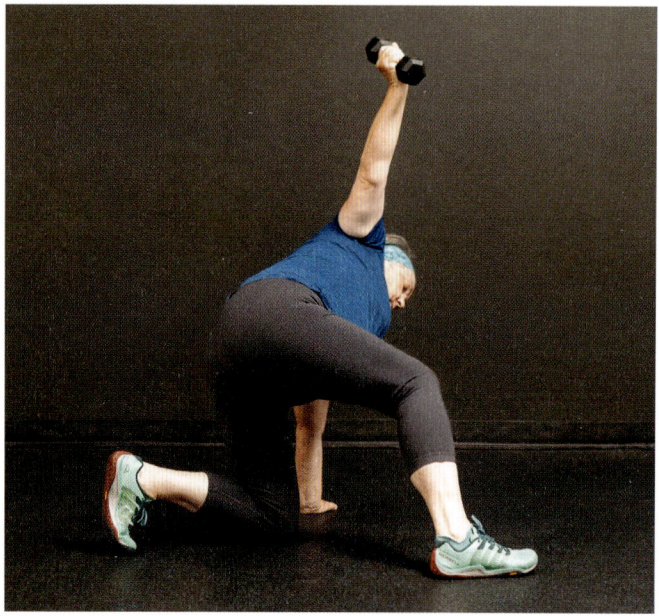

FIGURE 6.17.

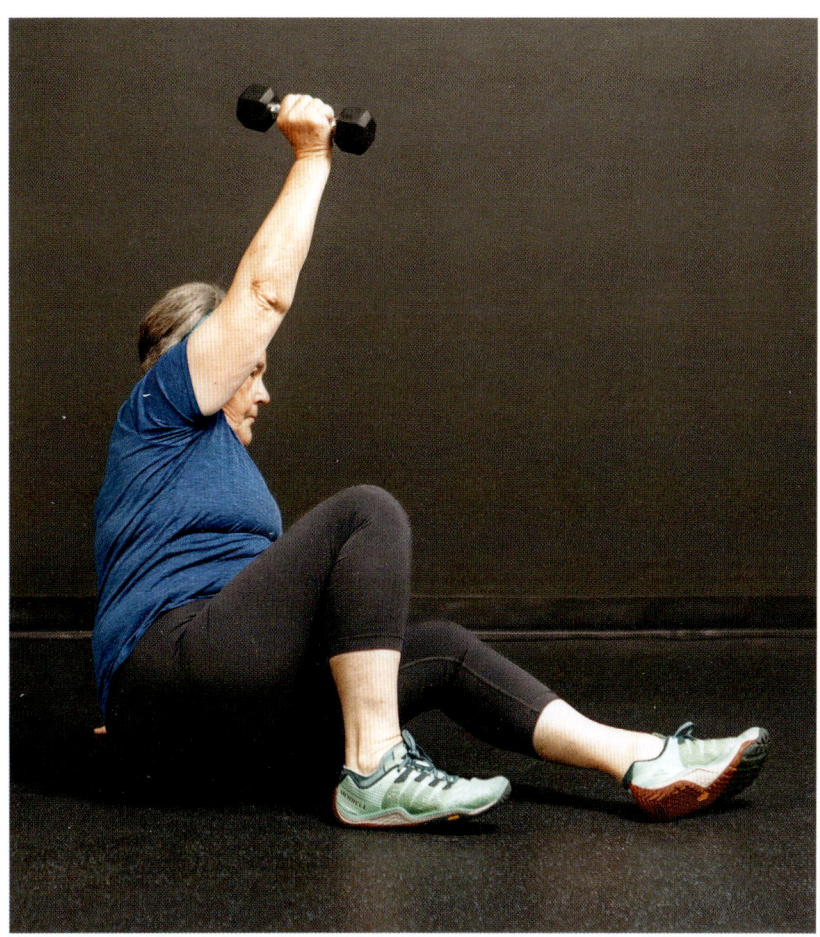

FIGURE 6.18.

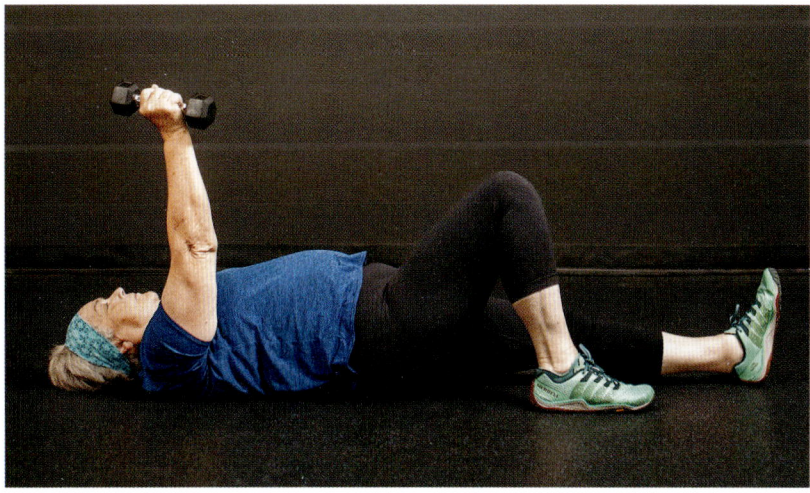

FIGURE 6.19.

REAL-LIFE SCENARIO: STANDING UP WHILE HOLDING A LOAD

This scenario simulates standing up from a seated position while carrying something like groceries or luggage, an everyday movement that we perform regularly. Let's break down the mechanics, first with a bag of groceries and then with carry-on luggage.

Here, the movement begins with Anthony seated tall but starting to rise. He is leaning forward slightly to initiate the lift.

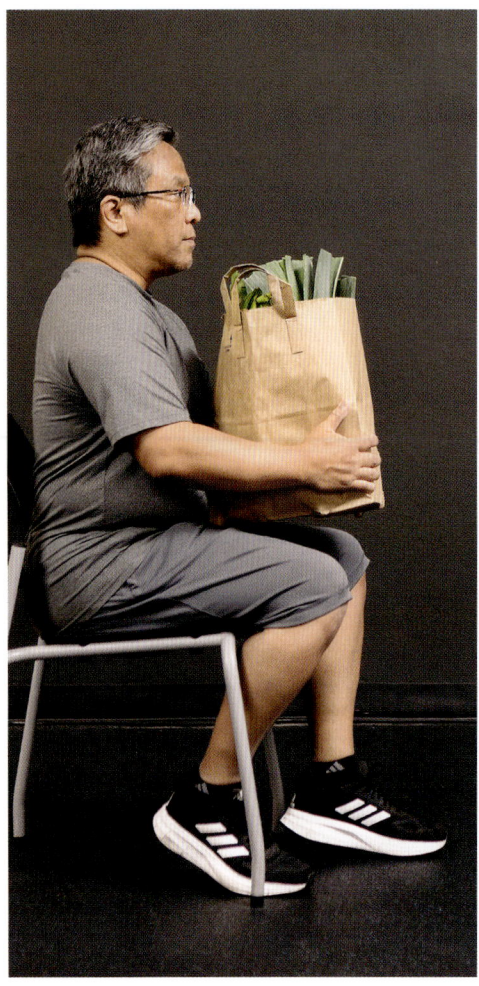 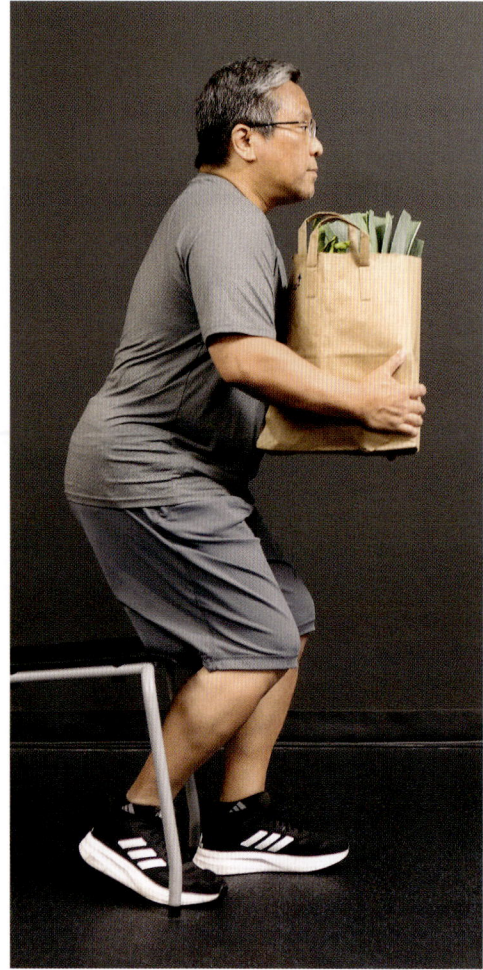

FIGURE 6.20.   **FIGURE 6.21.**

As Anthony rises, his legs are fully engaged, with his knees soft and slightly bent to stabilize the transition. His posture remains upright, and he keeps the weight close to his center of gravity for control.

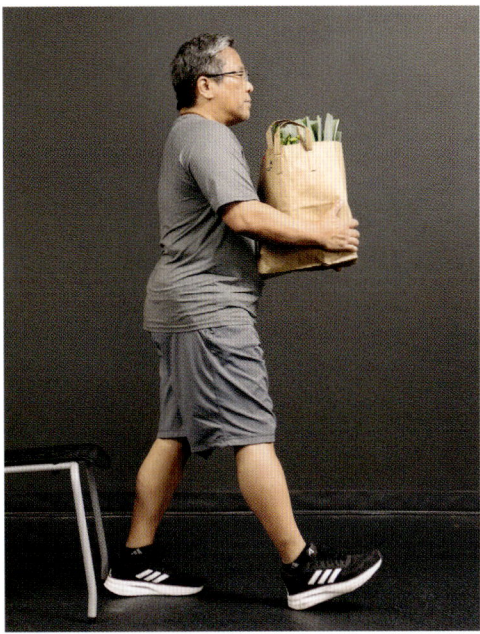

FIGURE 6.22.

The movement completes as he transitions to walking, demonstrating functional strength and balance.

The next sequence depicts a similar motion but with carry-on luggage held in one hand, emphasizing the asymmetry of the load.

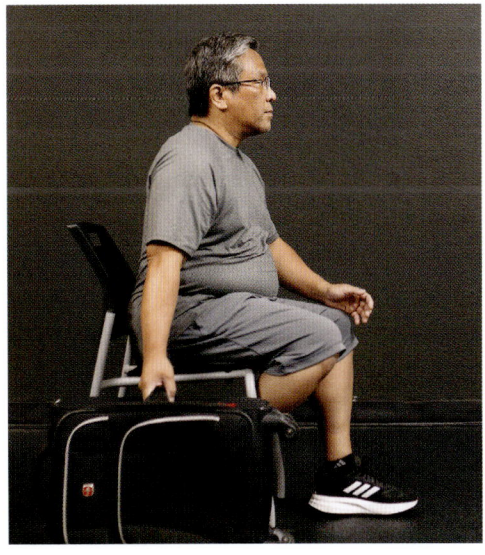

FIGURE 6.23.

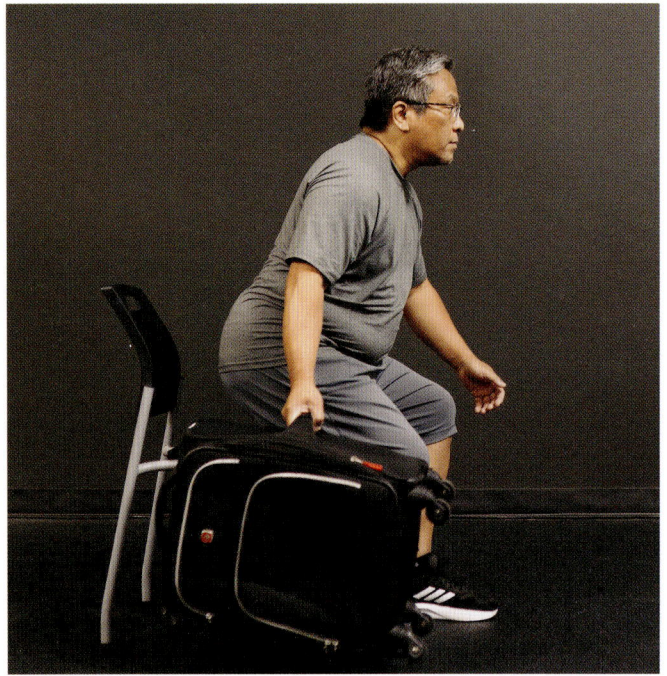

FIGURE 6.24.

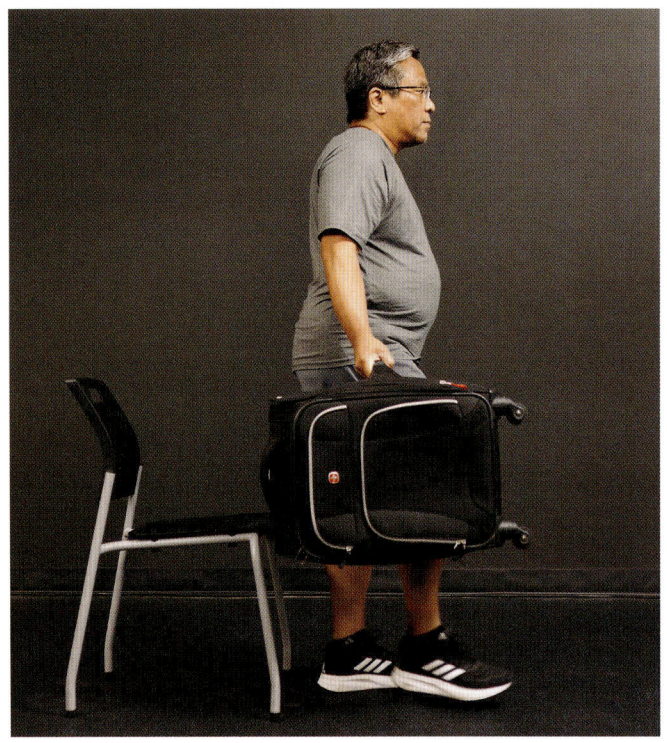

FIGURE 6.25.

What I See: These movements resemble a *squat performed with a weight*. As discussed earlier in this chapter, moving with external weight should be part of each squat exercise, given how often we do this daily. Let's look at a squat exercise that prepares us for these real-life scenarios, using asymmetrical weight (e.g., a single kettlebell or dumbbell) held in one hand. A squat can also be performed using evenly distributed weight held with both hands, but working with a weight in only one hand is important because we often carry things in one hand and aren't always perfectly balanced. This movement involves more than just holding the item—it works our core to keep our frame square and practices engaging one leg and hip more than the other.

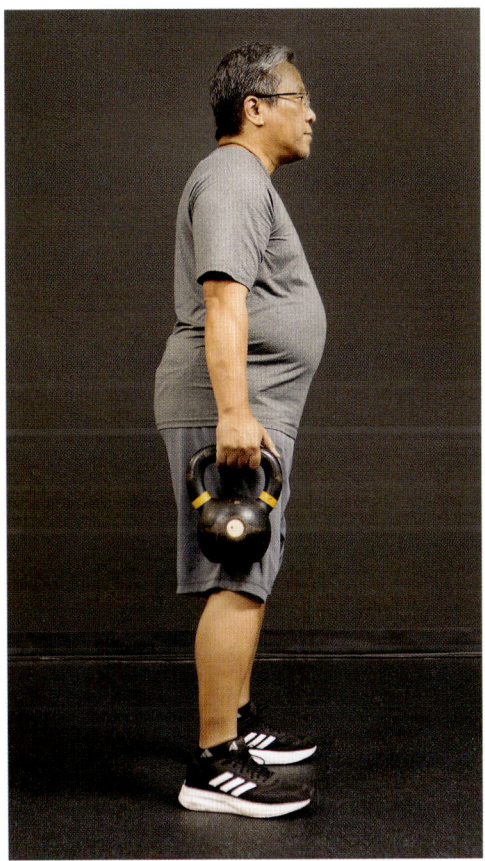

FIGURE 6.26.

Holding the kettlebell in one hand creates an imbalance, engaging the core to maintain posture.

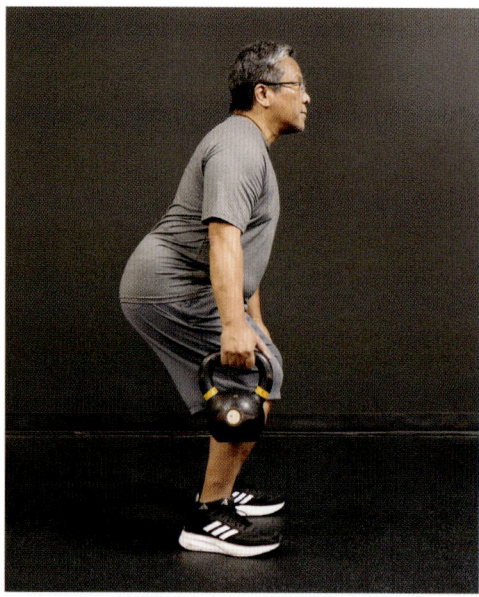

FIGURE 6.27.

As Anthony lowers into a squat, his legs and core work to stabilize the uneven load. His chest stays upright, and his hips move back in a controlled descent.

The following images provide a front view of the same movement, highlighting the need for equal effort from both sides of the body, even when the weight is held on one side.

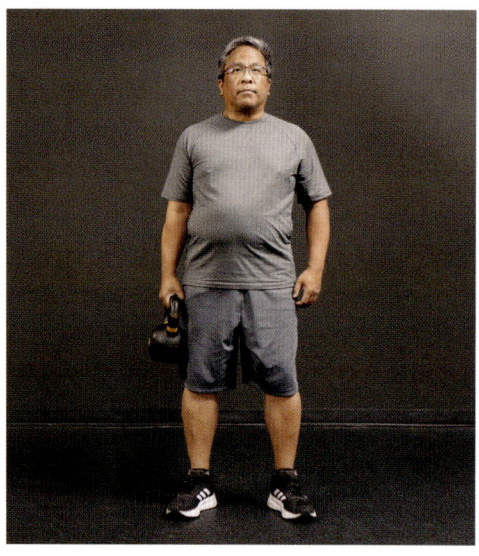

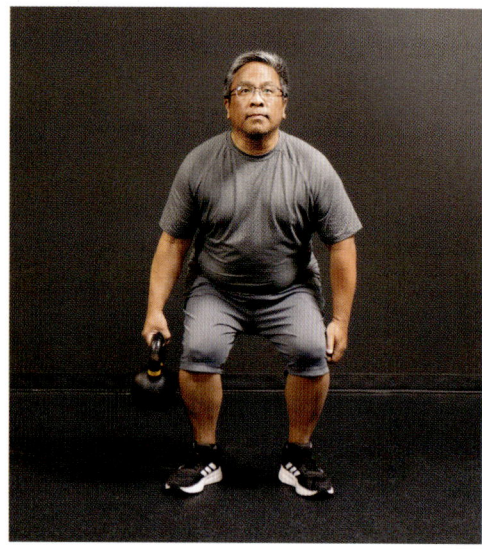

FIGURE 6.28.   **FIGURE 6.29.**

REAL-LIFE SCENARIO: MOVING GROCERIES OR HEAVY ITEMS

This scenario highlights common everyday movements like moving groceries out of your car, organizing heavy items, or in Ruth's case, setting up at the farmers market. Ruth's actions in this sequence depict picking up and moving objects from a table to the floor and vice versa.

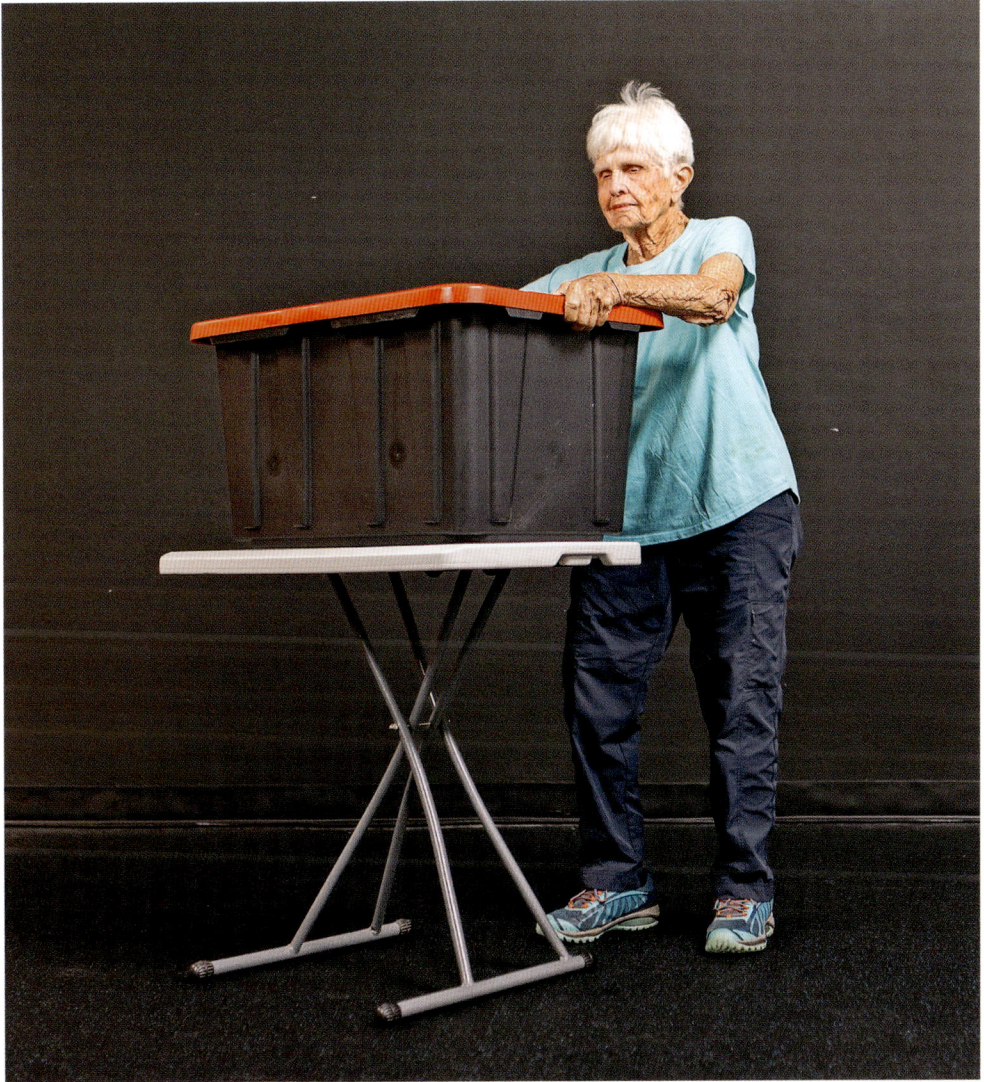

FIGURE 6.30.

Here, Ruth prepares to pick up the container by gripping it firmly with both hands, aligning her body for the lift.

She rotates her torso while keeping the container close to her body, engaging her core to maintain balance during the turn.

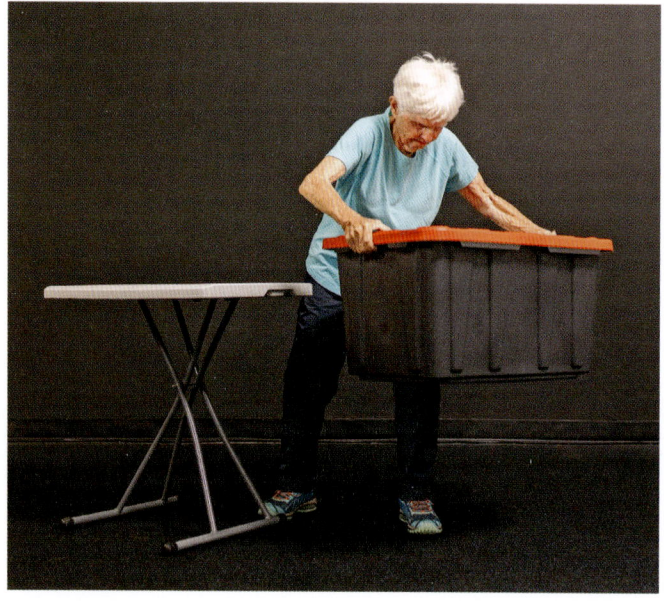

FIGURE 6.31.

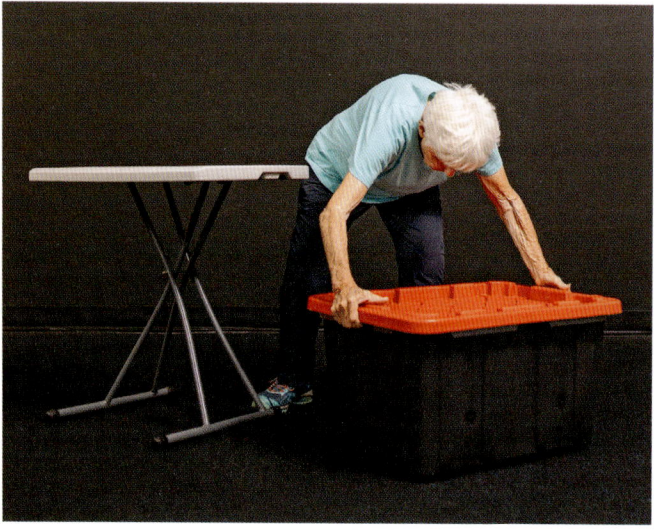

FIGURE 6.32.

She hinges her hips and bends her knees as she completes the motion, controlling the descent to avoid strain on her lower back.

What I See: This movement simply boils down to picking up heavy objects at a height and placing them on the ground or a lower surface using rotational motion. Notice the similarities to the next exercise sequence that involves picking up a weight from the ground and placing it back down. This type of rotational training incorporates controlled twisting motions into your routine, enhancing core strength and stability.

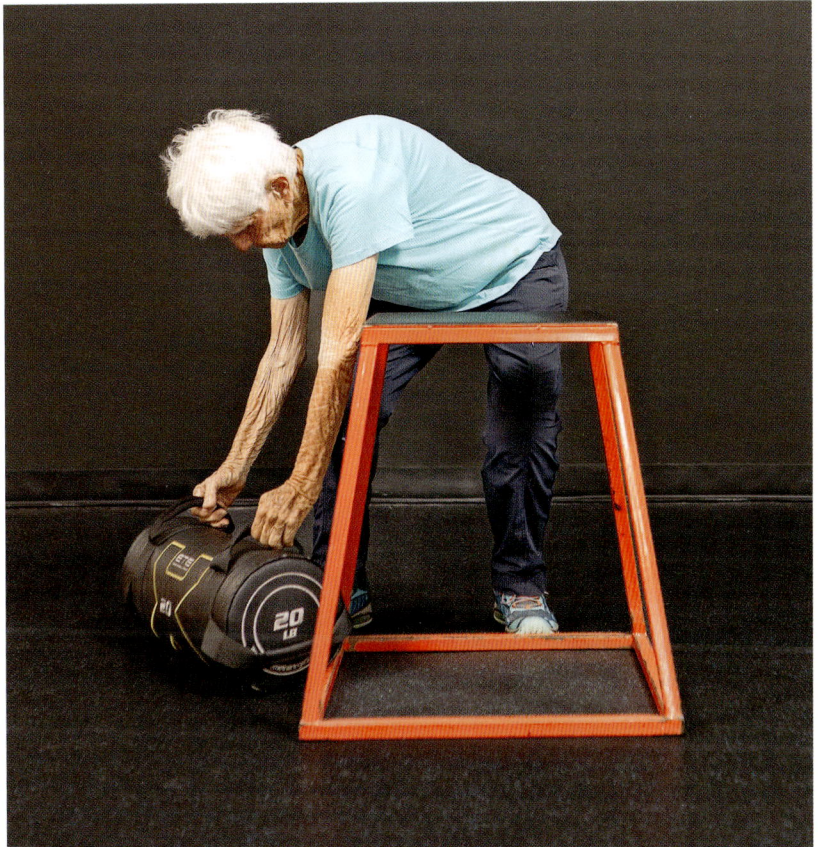

FIGURE 6.33.

When we pick up things, we often twist at the same time. Here, Ruth is hinging her hips back and lowering herself by bending her knees to pick up a sandbag. This is the safe way to pick up low-lying objects. She lifts by loading up her glutes and legs, rather than her back, which reduces the chances of injury. She also engages her core. Picking heavy objects off the ground is commonly called a *deadlift*. You will see the more standard versions of a deadlift a bit later in the chapter.

Rotational strength and coordination come into play as Ruth lifts and turns simultaneously, further engaging her shoulders, arms, and core.

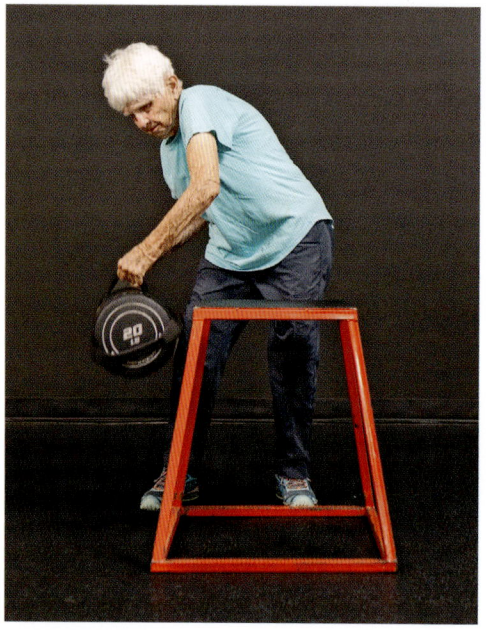

FIGURE 6.34.

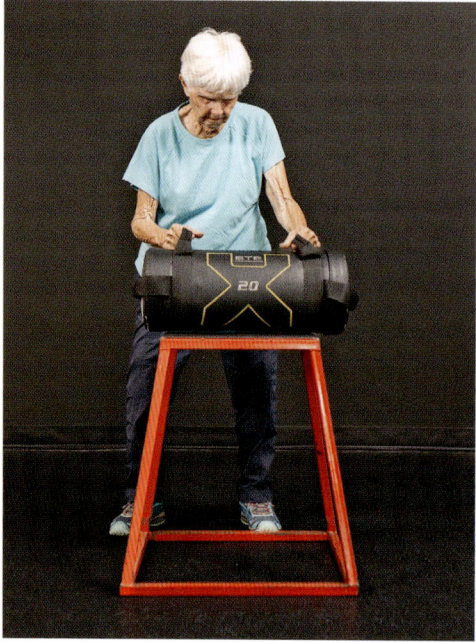

FIGURE 6.35.

Ruth completes the lift and places the sandbag on the bench by using her arms and shoulders to pull the weight toward herself. This exercise helps Ruth remain able to put her boxes from the market up on tables and into her truck.

In the following images, Ruth reverses the motion, using the same mechanics to lower the sandbag safely with control. She pulls the weight closer to herself and then hinges her hips back and reaches down, demonstrating a full-body movement that takes strength and coordination.

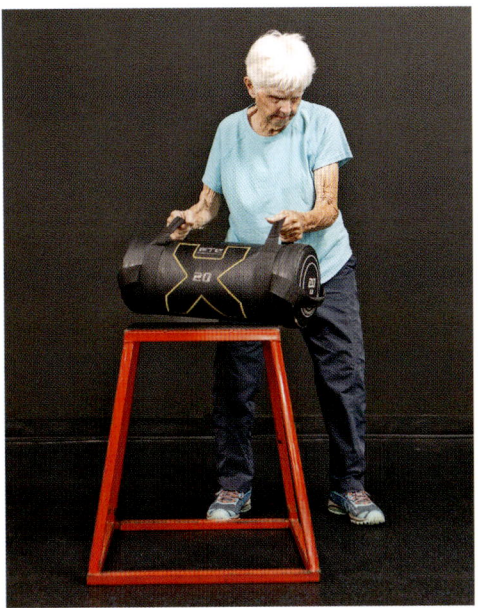

FIGURE 6.36.

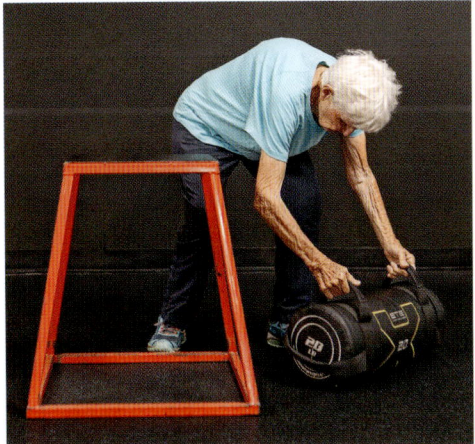

FIGURE 6.37.

REAL-LIFE SCENARIO: GRIPPING AND PULLING HEAVY LOADS DURING YARD WORK OR CHORES

Yard work and other household chores often require pulling movements combined with grip strength. In this scenario, the heavy bags of soil are too large and heavy to lift conventionally, using a squat or deadlift form, so they must be moved by pulling. This action requires tightly grasping the load, core bracing (using core strength for stability while pulling), and controlled backpedals to avoid low back injury.

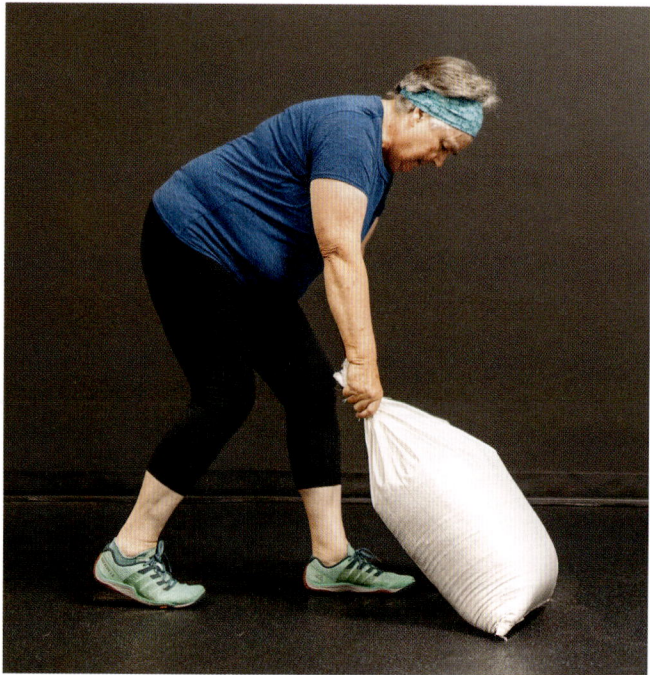

FIGURE 6.38.

Here, Martha tightly grips the top of the bag and pulls it while engaging her core and using her legs to backpedal. Her low back remains neutral to avoid strain.

What I See: *Rows.* These build upper-body strength, aiding in lifting and pulling motions. There are many ways to practice the pulling motion of rowing. In the following sequence, Martha demonstrates a *suspension row*, which uses a suspension tool. One of the hidden benefits of this exercise is that it develops grip strength. While this gym workout does not perfectly mirror real-life situations like setting up a tent or opening a picnic table, the movements in both settings involve pulling and using grip strength to accomplish the actions. Martha uses her core strength through a technique known in fitness as bracing—essentially, she engages the muscles around her spine to create the stability needed to pull efficiently. Bracing is often described as how you would engage your core if you knew someone would punch you in the stomach. As Martha braces, her hip muscles likely engage as well to keep her feet squarely planted and allow her arms to go to work.

The position in figure 6.39 is the starting point for Martha's suspension rows. The straight-line posture engages the core muscles to stabilize her body, preventing sagging or overextension. The grip strength needed to hold the straps mimics the real-life need for a firm grasp when pulling.

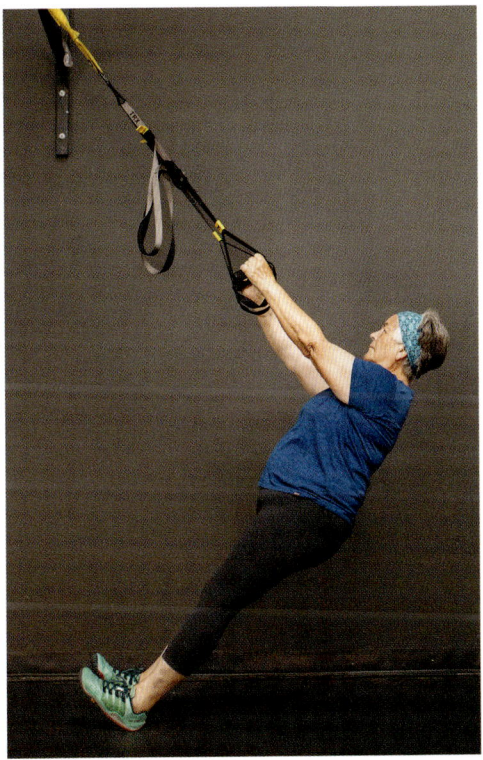 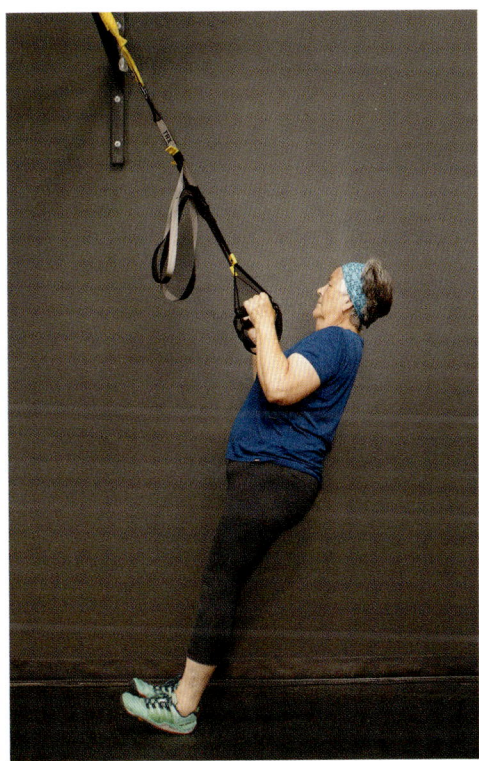

FIGURE 6.39.   **FIGURE 6.40.**

In this phase (figure 6.40), her arms, shoulders, and back muscles perform the pulling action. Her core remains braced to maintain stability, and her feet act as the anchor point, much like when pulling a heavy object in real life.

REAL-LIFE SCENARIO: PICKING UP SOMETHING HEAVY

We encounter this scenario frequently in everyday life when lifting a heavy object like a bag of soil, a heavy bag of groceries, or, as in this example, a full five-gallon water bottle. Let's examine some key movements and how they translate to specific exercises.

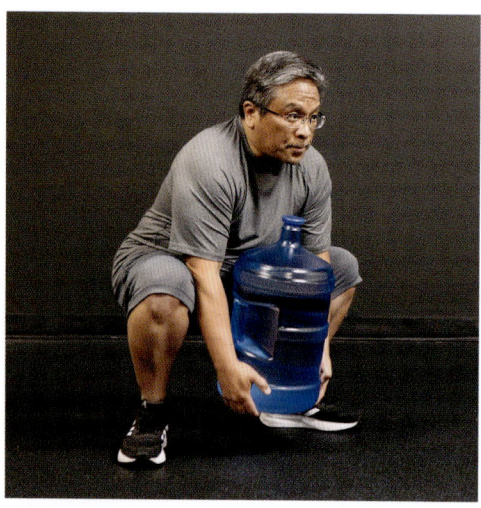

FIGURE 6.41.

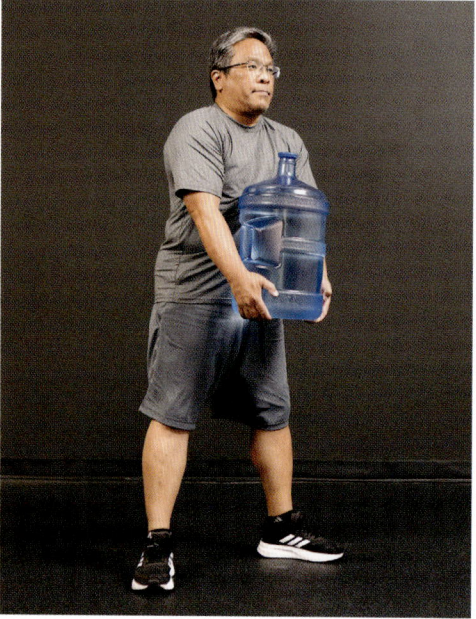

FIGURE 6.42.

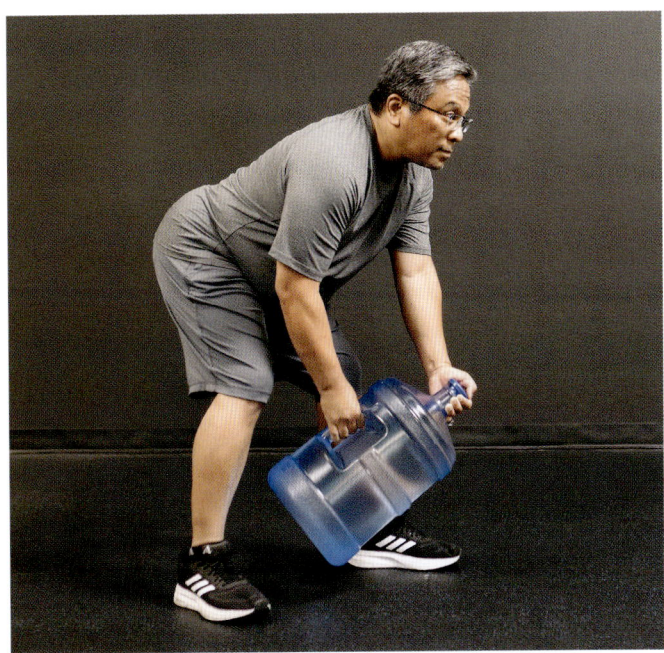

FIGURE 6.43.

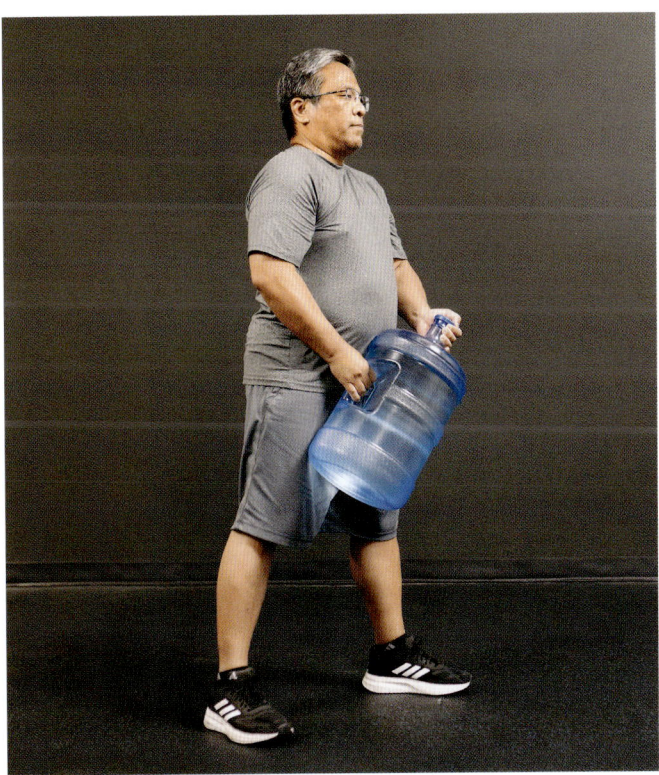

FIGURE 6.44.

What I See: I see two ways of picking something up—using a squat or a deadlift movement. The squat, as we've seen in the earlier scenario, focuses on leg, glute, and core strength. Adding a weight further challenges the body by also working the arms and grip for full-body engagement. Squat movements are helpful for tasks where the heavy object can be held close to the body while being lifted from or placed down on the ground or in a low position. For proper form, the back should remain straight, the core must activate to stabilize the movement, and the weight should be held close to minimize strain on the lower back and spine. Holding a heavier weight, similar to the kettlebell used in the squat sequence earlier, is a good way to practice this.

Let's now focus on the other way Anthony picks the bottle up, which is complemented by practicing a *deadlift with a barbell*.

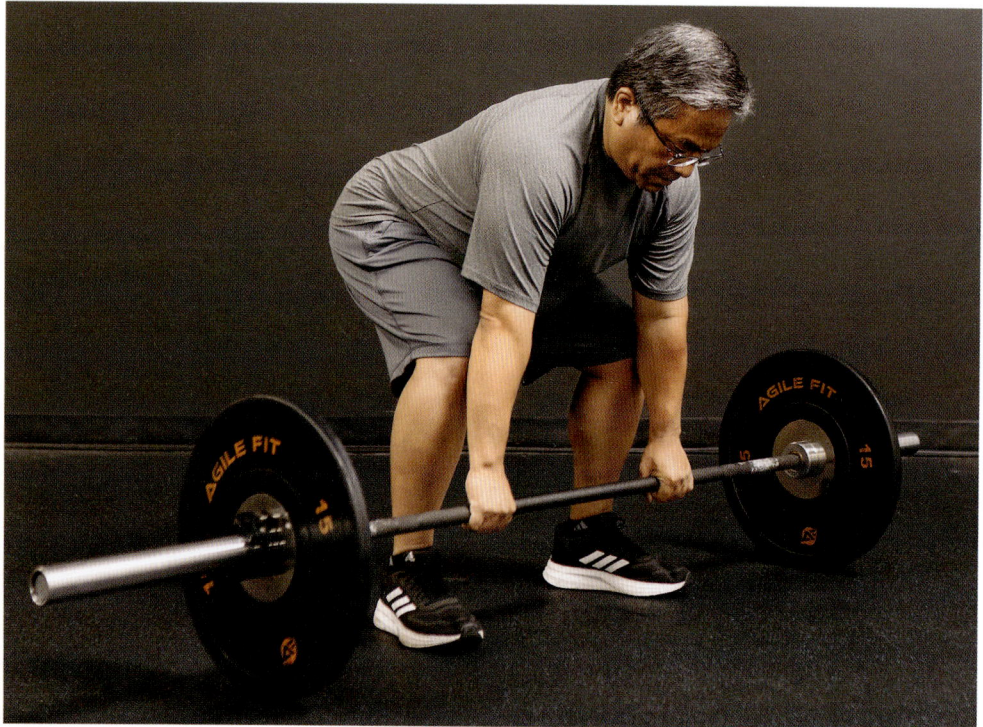

FIGURE 6.45.

This starting position is critical and mirrors the initial position for picking up the water bottle with a deadlift movement. His hips are back, knees bent, back flat, and arms straight as he leans forward. The barbell is placed close to his body to reduce strain on the lower back.

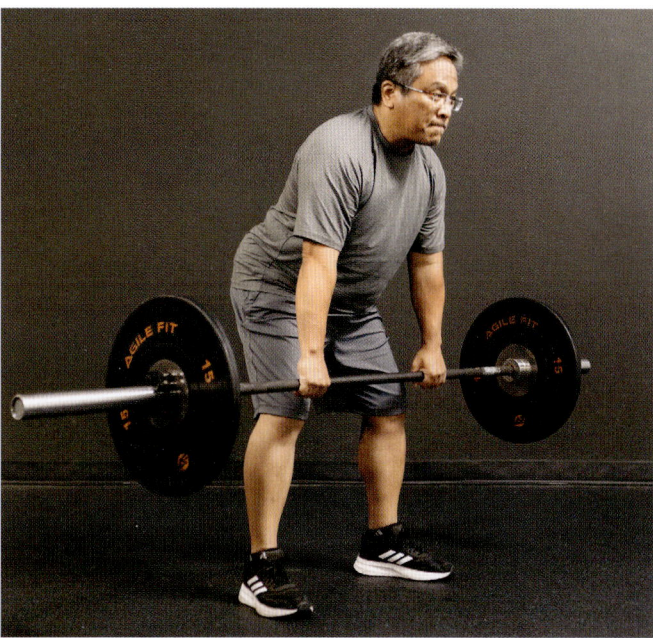

FIGURE 6.46.

As Anthony lifts the barbell, he visualizes putting his feet through the floor and engages his leg muscles and glutes to stand up while his core remains braced for stability. Notice how the barbell remains close to his body.

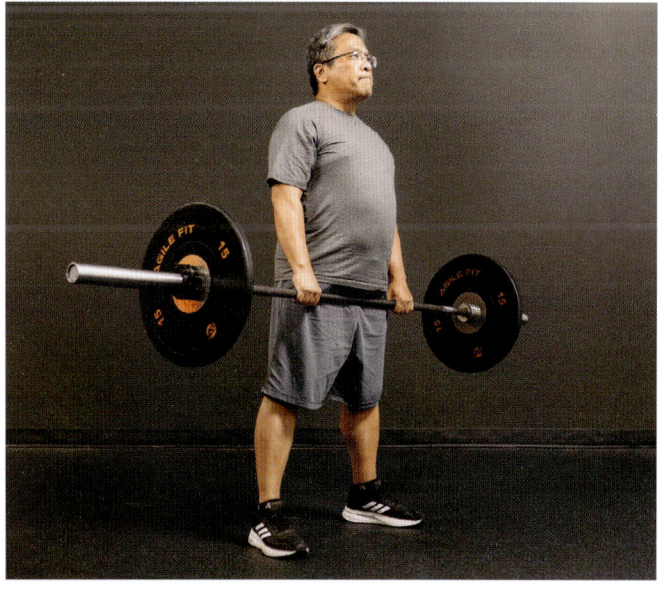

FIGURE 6.47.

This final position emphasizes standing tall with proper posture. His shoulders are square and his grip, core, and lower body work together to stabilize the barbell. This phase mirrors the standing position when lifting a heavy object like the water bottle in real life.

Performing a deadlift to lift a heavy weight from the ground strengthens the body from head to toe, engaging the muscles of the legs, glutes, core, back, arms (including hands and wrists for grip strength), and trapezius. This exercise reminds us to follow key principles when lifting heavy objects: Keep the weight close to effectively place the load on the legs and glutes and avoid hurting our back; brace the core for stability; use legs and glutes to lift; keep a straight back to avoid rounding the spine; and maintain a firm grip to secure the weight. For optimal deadlift technique, you should be able to draw a relatively straight line from your shoulder, through the bar, to your foot throughout the movement, as seen in these images.

REAL-LIFE SCENARIO: LIFTING AND PLACING ITEMS OVERHEAD

Lifting and placing things on a high shelf or on top of the fridge is a common activity in everyday life. The following example demonstrates putting carry-on luggage in an airplane's overhead bin. Let's break down the movement and examine how it translates to specific exercises.

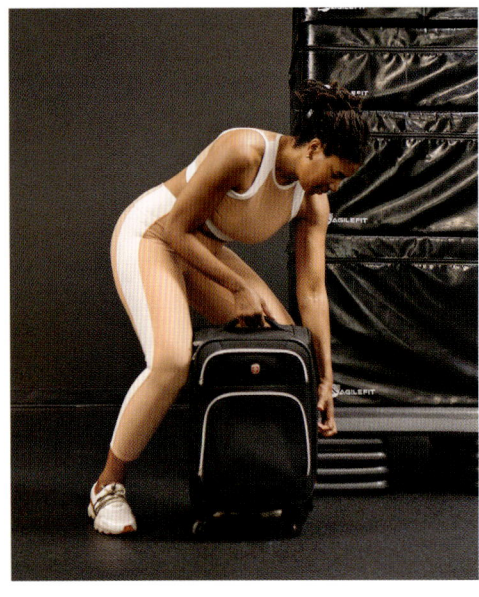

FIGURE 6.48. **FIGURE 6.49.**

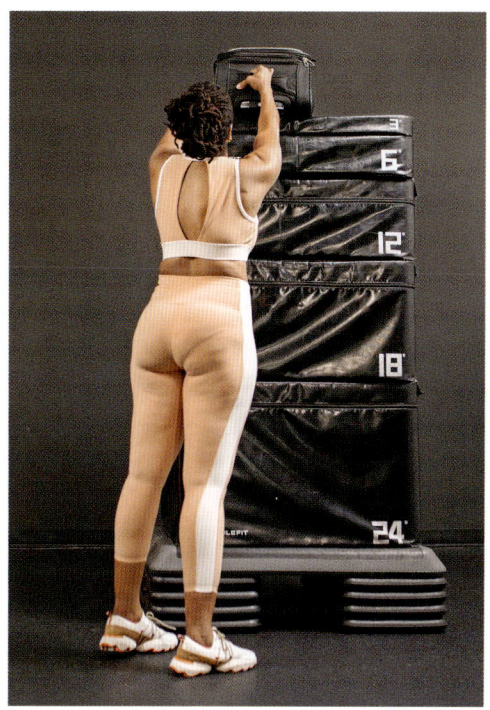

FIGURE 6.50.

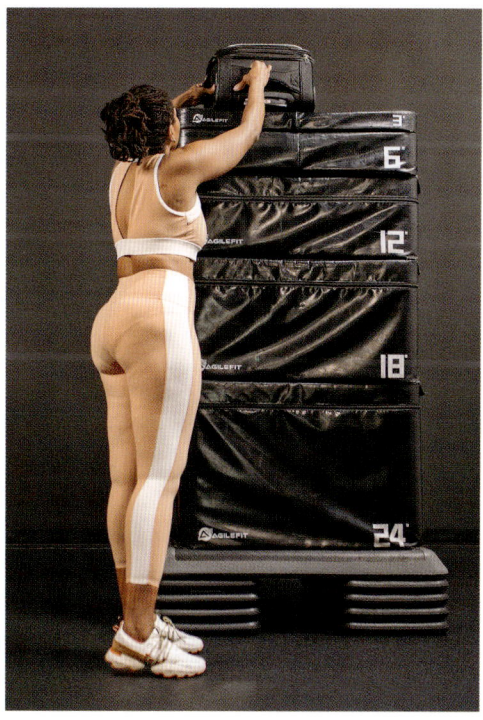

FIGURE 6.51.

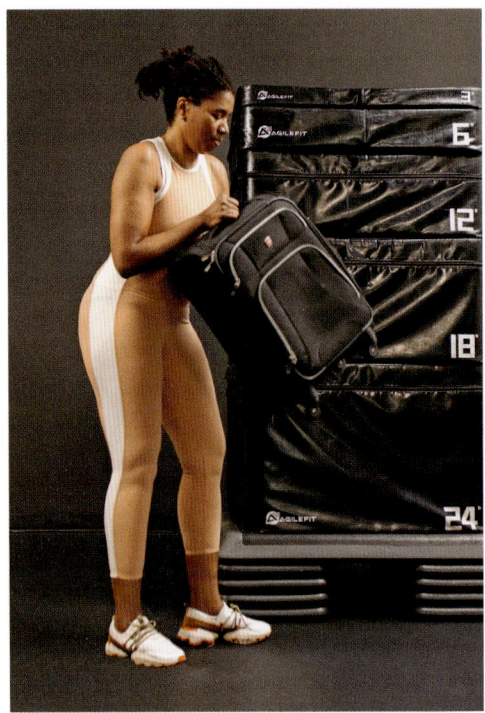

FIGURE 6.52.

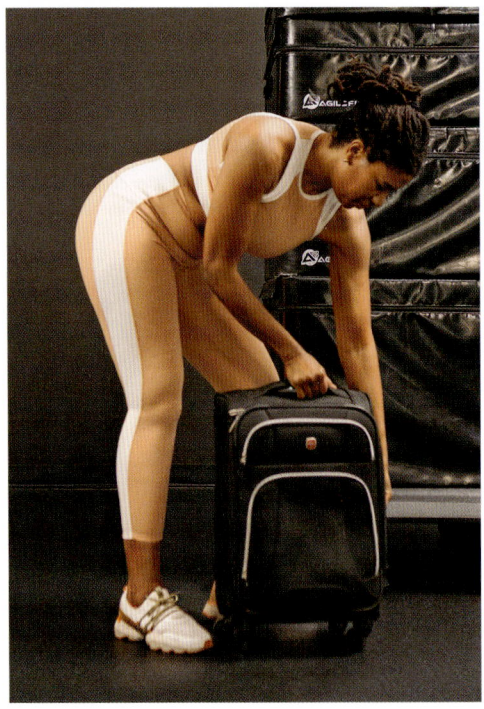

FIGURE 6.53.

What I See: Picking up a heavy object from the ground and placing it over-head, as well as the reverse action of lowering it back to the ground, involves the entire body. A few significant exercises hidden in Debra's movements include: rows, a squat to press, and a deadlift. Again, I urge you not to think these movements are beyond your ability. The amount of weight and the exercise tools you use while performing these movements may differ, but you can and should do some variation of each of them. Let's consider these three exercises in more detail.

In figures 6.54 to 6.57, we see Debra performing *double dumbbell rows*. This exercise strengthens the arm, shoulder, and upper back muscles. The flat-back posture required for this movement also engages the core muscles. All of these muscle groups are essential for pulling heavy objects toward the body. Maintaining a flat back during this exercise is crucial to prevent back strain and injury. Practicing this movement reinforces good posture and pulling mechanics, both of which are important for safely handling heavy objects, whether in the gym or during everyday activities.

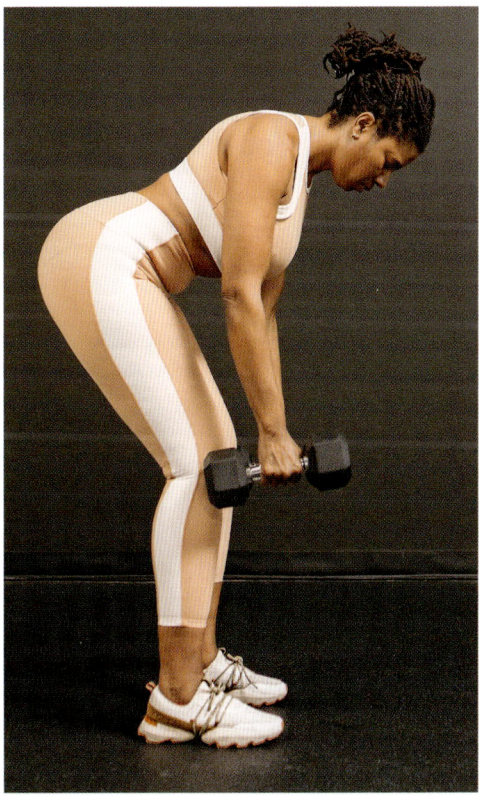

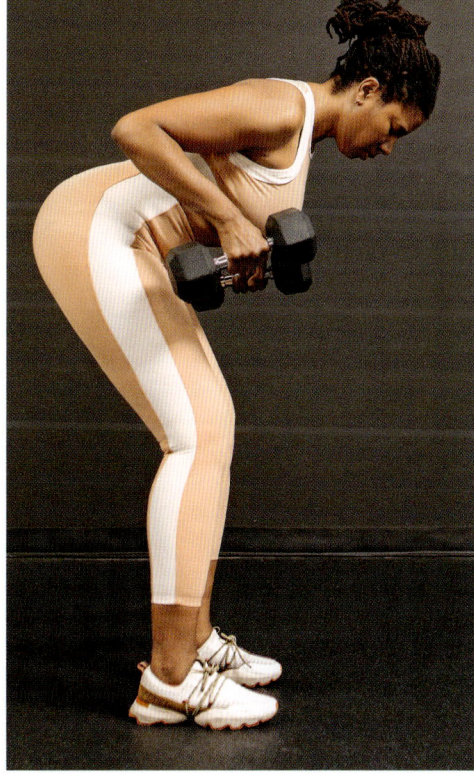

FIGURE 6.54.　　　　　　　　**FIGURE 6.55.**

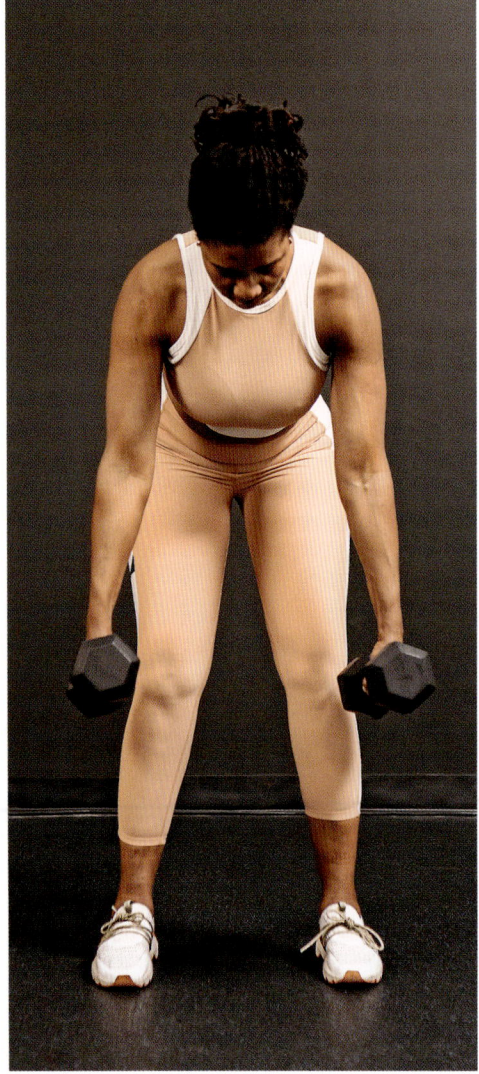

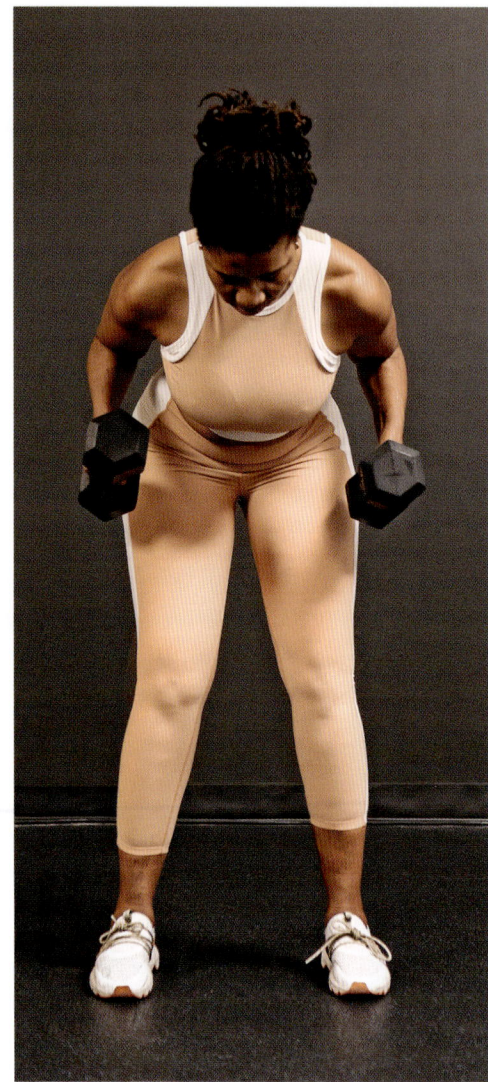

FIGURE 6.56.   **FIGURE 6.57.**

The *squat to press* (figures 6.58 and 6.59) combines lower-body strength (squatting) with upper-body power (pressing). It works the legs, core, shoulders, and arms in a coordinated way. Figures 6.58 and 6.59 show Debra performing this exercise with the ViPR PRO®, a cylindrical exercise tool that is particularly useful. Its handles facilitate grasping and keeping the tool level while pressing it overhead. Because this equipment is weighted (at eight kilograms), holding it helps build grip strength and forces the small stabilizer muscles in the shoulders and arms to work harder to maintain control.

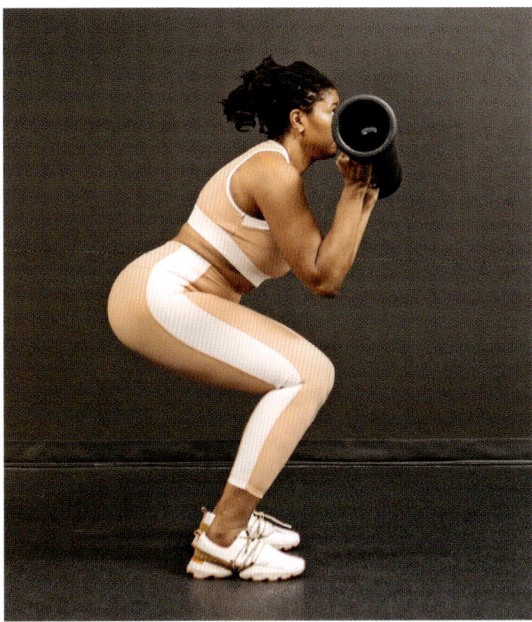

FIGURE 6.58.

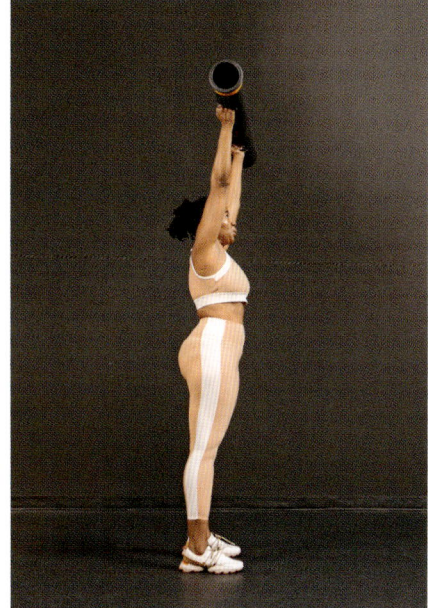

FIGURE 6.59.

In figures 6.60 and 6.61, we see Debra performing a *deadlift* with a different bar from the barbell used in the previous deadlift sequence (in the five-gallon water bottle series). This bar is called a hex bar. However, the execution and overall benefits remain the same.

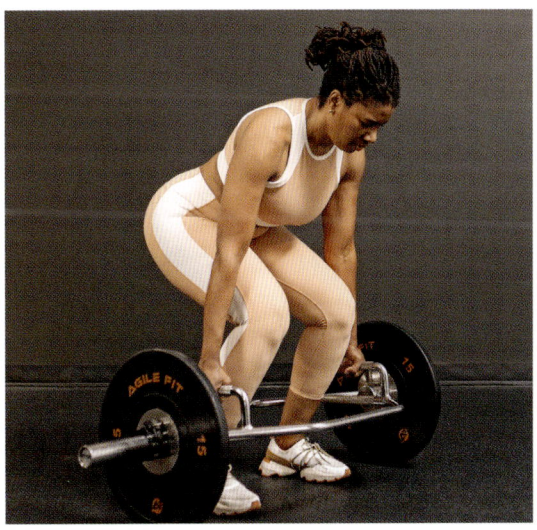
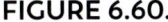

FIGURE 6.60.

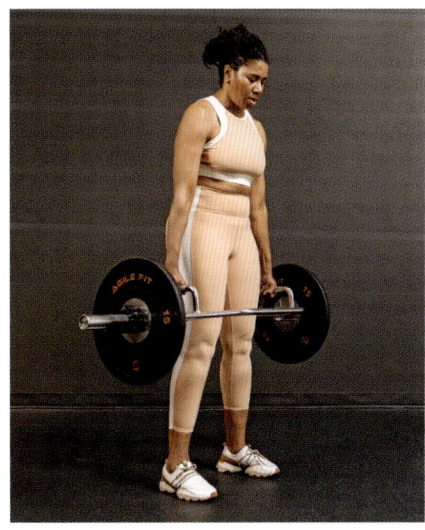

FIGURE 6.61.

Putting it all together . . .

Lifting something heavy, like luggage, into an overhead bin or shelf involves a coordinated sequence of movements that can be considered a full-body exercise, particularly when the luggage weighs close to the 22 lb. limit set by most airlines. Picking that weight up may be easy for some but having the power to lift it overhead is a whole other story. Here's how each exercise contributes to this real-life scenario:

- **Rows.** This exercise prepares the shoulders, arms, and upper back to pull the luggage toward your body, whether from the ground or a table.

- **Squat to press.** This movement strengthens the legs and core to squat with stability while simultaneously building the muscles of the upper body to press the luggage overhead. It also improves overall balance during overhead pressing.

- **Deadlifts.** This exercise helps us call on the right muscles to safely lift luggage off the ground. Instead of relying on our back for the lifting motion, we learn to hinge at the hips and use our legs, glutes, and core while also engaging our shoulders and back. Practicing this movement also reminds us to keep the weight close to our body to reduce back strain.

All three movements build grip strength, reinforce core engagement, and teach how to activate the back while keeping it flat to protect it from injury. They also help train the body to bring heavy objects back down safely and with control.

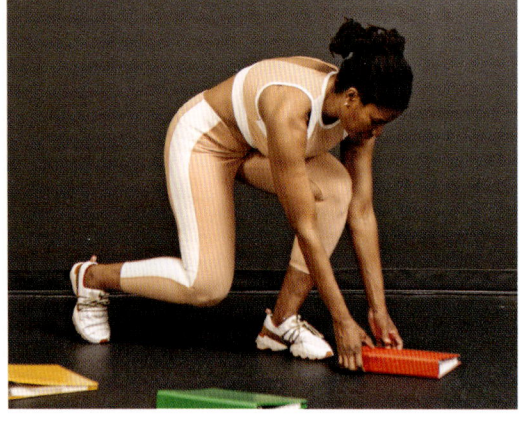

FIGURE 6.62.

REAL-LIFE SCENARIO: PICKING UP SMALL OBJECTS FROM THE FLOOR

We all encounter situations where we need to bend down and pick up small objects like toys, trash, or spilled groceries from a bag that has split open. In this instance, Debra's task involves retrieving a few binders scattered on the ground. There are many ways to accomplish this, as illustrated by the images here.

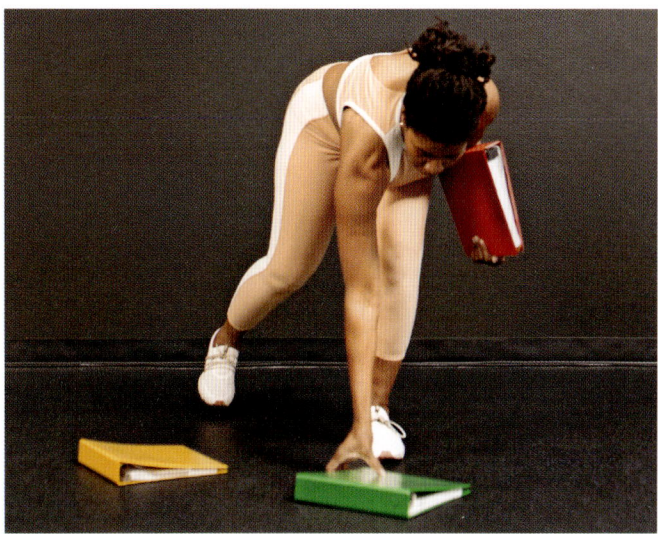

FIGURE 6.63.

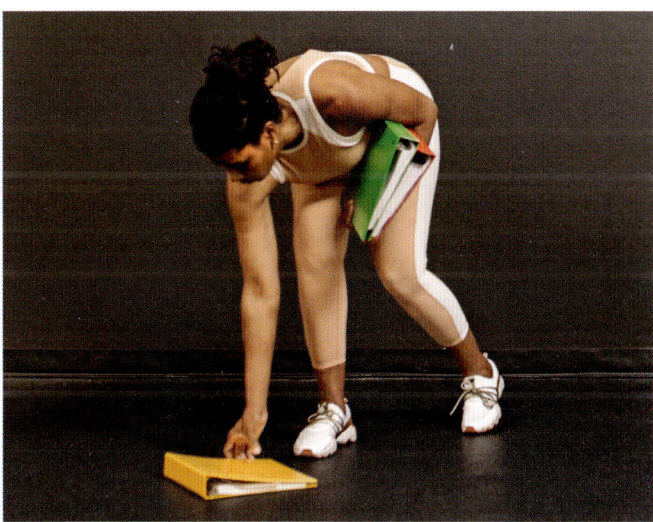

FIGURE 6.64.

What I See: *Lunges.* In everyday life, lunges are rarely performed in a precise way. Real-life movements often involve shifting weight, bending at different angles, and moving dynamically to retrieve objects that are spread out. In the gym, however, lunges are typically practiced in a straight line—whether they are rear, lateral, forward, or diagonal lunges. Remember that in the gym, we focus on more difficult movements to make our real-life movements easier. To increase the challenge, these controlled movements are often paired with weights or other variations, such as pushing a ball away from the body or hitting multiple angles. Fitness professionals also emphasize "sinking into" the lunge to effectively engage the glutes.

Let's break down how practicing lunges can prepare you for real-world tasks.

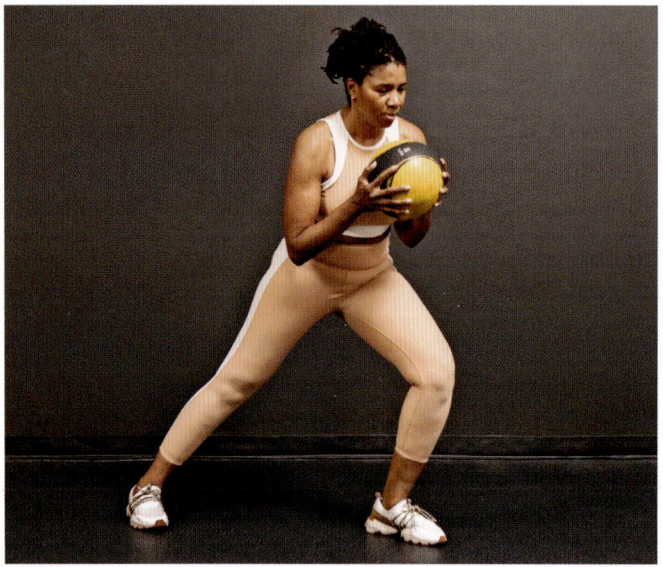

FIGURE 6.65.

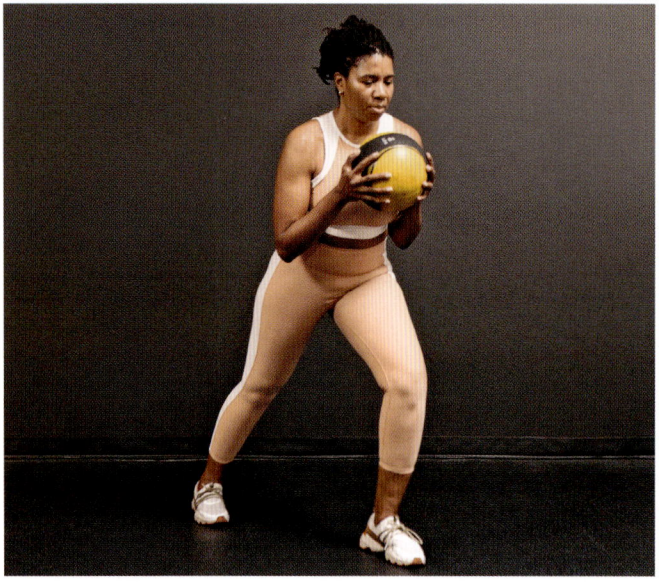

FIGURE 6.66.

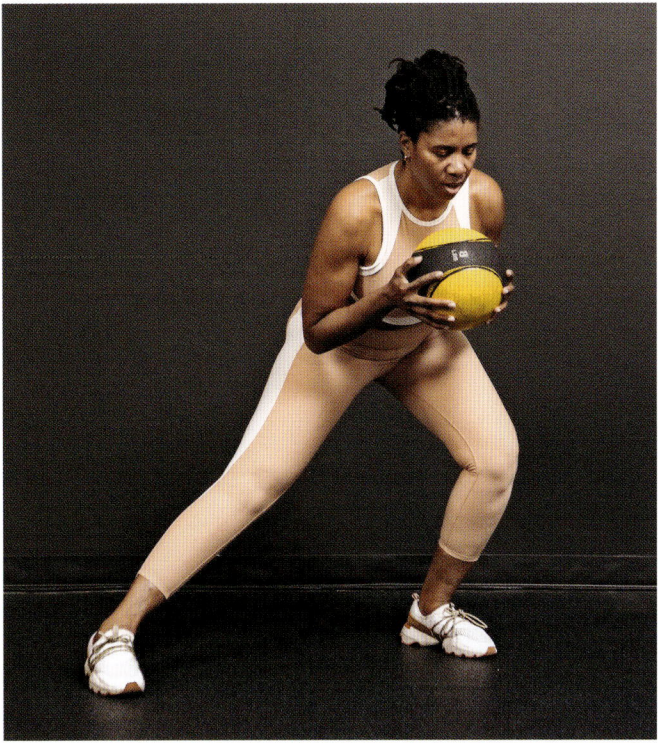

FIGURE 6.67.

One of the ways lunges help is that they train you to shift your weight when picking up objects from the floor. Although your feet stay on the ground during lunges, each variation requires moving in different directions, which shifts your weight accordingly. This process challenges your balance in the background and improves coordination. Additionally, one leg does more work to stabilize and support your weight during the movement, enhancing unilateral strength. This is crucial for real-life moments when one leg bears more load, such as when you lean forward or to the side to pick something up.

REAL-LIFE SCENARIO: YARD WORK

Yard work, in its many forms, requires moving in different directions and can be a full-body workout. For example, consider raking. Debris, such as leaves or soil, acts as an external weight being pulled toward you as you rake. The more the debris, the more effort is needed to gather it. Consequently, as the workload increases, so does the strength required to rake effectively. Also, it is essential to maintain a strong grip on the rake handle, especially as the load becomes heavier or when you speed up your raking tempo.

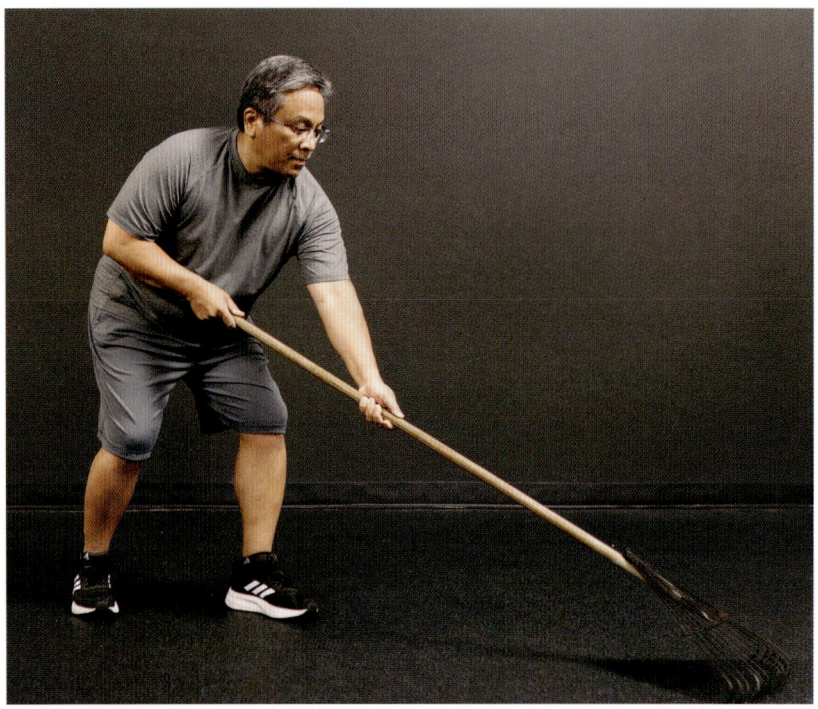

FIGURE 6.68.

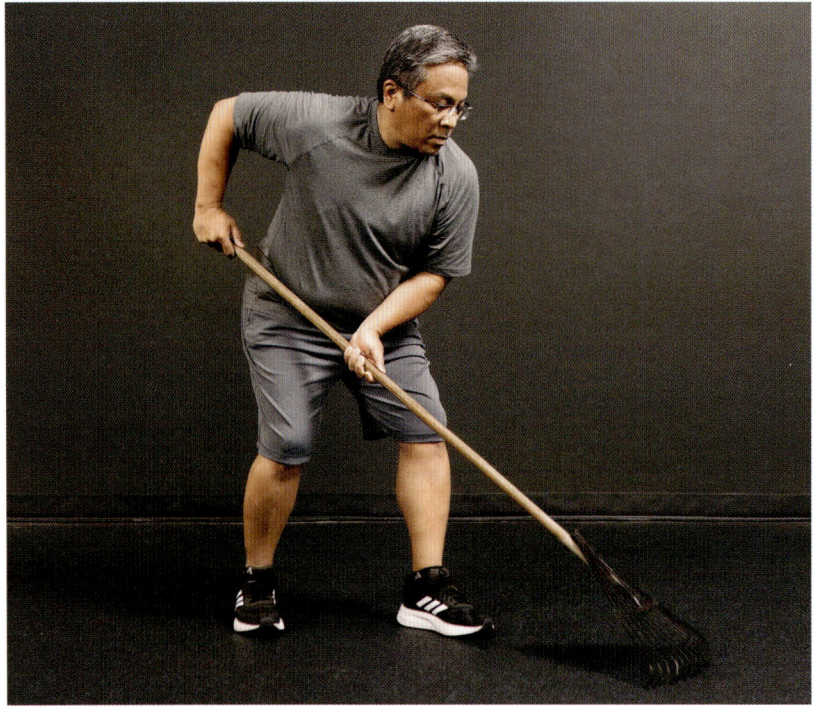

FIGURE 6.69.

What I See: *Core Strength.* This movement demands arm strength, core strength, and stability. In the half-kneeling exercise known as the *Pallof press,* shown in figures 6.70 to 6.72, Anthony exerts substantial effort to maintain proper form. There is significant tension in the resistance band, which tries to pull him off balance. To counter this, he must keep his core engaged and rely on the stability of his hips to own the position. As he turns, even with his arms extended, he engages his back and core muscles to uphold a tall posture. This exercise, when combined with deadlifts, helps ensure a secure grip on the rake handle and promotes an upright posture from hips to shoulders—without rounding the back.

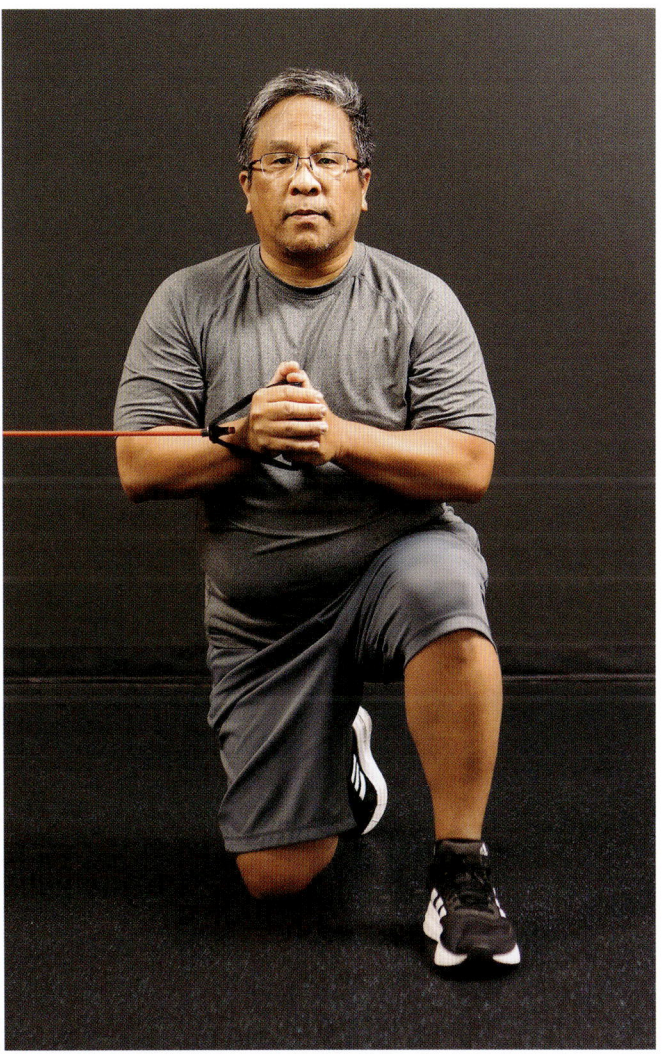

FIGURE 6.70.

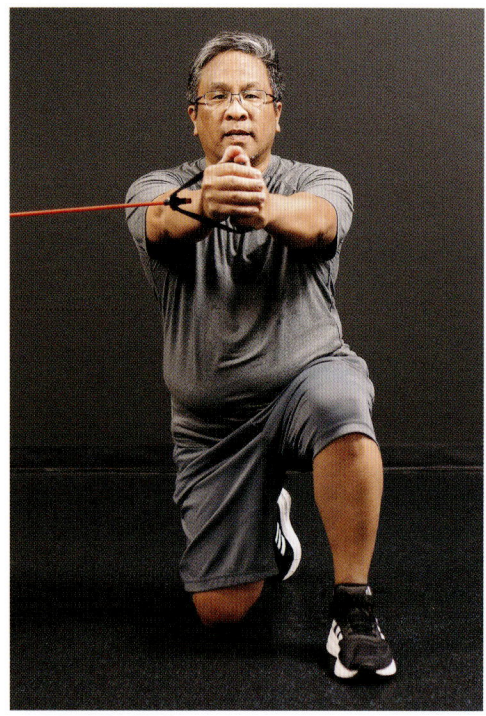

FIGURE 6.71.

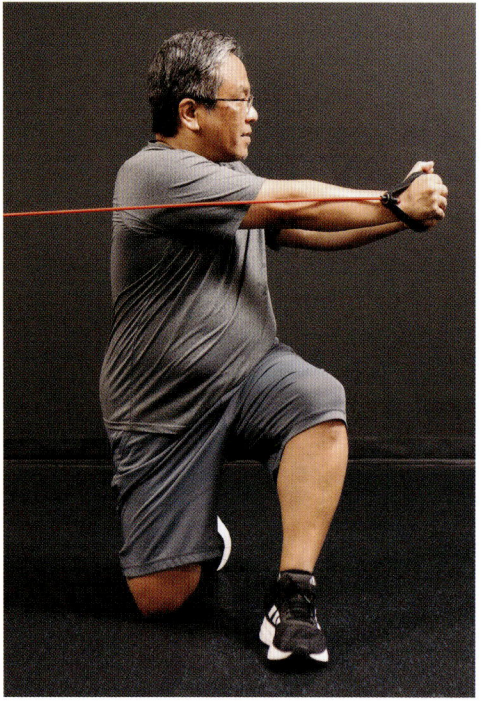

FIGURE 6.72.

* * *

As you can see, real-life activities do not always involve perfectly measured weights, flat surfaces, or predictable environments. When we practice better and more optimal movement in an exercise setting, we can transfer those skills to real-life situations. This not only makes everyday life safer and more manageable but also enables you to move with confidence.

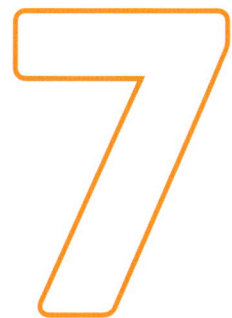

PRACTICE MAKES BETTER

> *Aging is an extraordinary process where you become the person you always should have been.*
>
> —DAVID BOWIE, *DAVID BOWIE: THE LAST INTERVIEW AND OTHER CONVERSATIONS*

Perfection? There is no such thing. Nature is beautifully imperfect, just like we are. And that imperfection is what makes life interesting. When it comes to movement and exercise, I argue against striving for perfection. Instead, strive to move better. Strive to improve, no matter how minuscule that improvement may be. Improvement is not about being perfect; it is about practicing to move better. Mistakes are an essential part of that process.

If sports are your thing, think about practice during the offseason. What do your favorite athletes do in the offseason? They work on performing better in their sport. They do strength training to improve their ability to move. They practice dynamic running drills to develop their ability to change direction quickly. Now imagine if a major football star spends the offseason just playing golf, partying late often, and eating poorly. How do you think they will perform on game day? Not great, that is for sure. The same goes for you. What you eat, how you move, and how you treat your body will directly affect your ability to move. For instance, if you spend the day having fast food and sugary drinks, you likely won't feel your best, mentally or physically. The key difference for you is that every day is game day. Some days may be more physically demanding than others, but every day, you still need to get out of bed. Every day, you pick up, move, and place down things. You sit down to use the bathroom. You reach for things around you. Ideally, all these movements should be performed with little to no discomfort.

Remember when we deputized you as a trainer a few chapters ago? Time to put that hat back on. Here's the scenario:

Don is a new client who has been training with you for just two weeks. His knees are generally okay, but he experiences knee pain during squats. Thanks to your experience, you notice that Don's squat form is putting too much pressure on his knees. You see that he needs to adjust his technique to shift more weight to his hamstrings and glutes. You also notice that when Don gets out of a chair, he rocks back and forth to generate enough momentum to stand. For today's workout, you have him do twelve squats as part of a routine that he will repeat three times. He is mildly interested but hesitant because he does not want to hurt his knees. He says he trusts you. What do you do?

A. Ask Don to do the squats while giving him various cues the entire time to help him achieve perfect form.

B. Stop Don every time he makes a mistake.

C. Give Don two or three key cues to improve his squat form, allow him to complete the set, and then provide additional feedback. Experiment with adjustments, such as changing his foot position, to see what works best for him.

D. Remove squats from Don's workout altogether because it is clear his form needs a lot of work, which will take effort and time.

Let's eliminate the options that aren't effective.

- **Option D.** Removing squats from the workout is not ideal. Don must sit down and stand up daily, so practicing this movement is essential. Just because there is room for improvement doesn't mean he can't make progress. Avoiding squats will not help him move better; instead, look for ways to modify the movement and improve his form.

- **Option B.** Stopping Don every time he makes a mistake would lead to frustration for both of you. He could lose confidence, feel overwhelmed, or become discouraged from continuing.

- **Option A.** Giving constant cues during every repetition could overwhelm Don by providing too much information. When concentrating on learning a movement, a constant stream of corrections can be too much to process and do all at once.

This leaves us with option C as the best approach. This option strikes the right balance. By giving Don two or three key cues to focus on, you avoid overwhelming him with overcoaching while allowing him to complete the set. Afterward, you can provide corrections and explore modifications to find what works best for him. This approach gives Don a chance to figure things out on his own during his set, allowing him to learn and progress without feeling rushed or pressured to be "perfect." Practice makes progress, and this approach helps him practice in a way that sets him up for success.

When you are your own trainer, remember to allow yourself to practice. Be patient with the process and recognize that learning to move better is just as much a mental journey as it is a physical one. I often see clients rediscover their bodies during our sessions. They become aware of tightness, limited range of motion, pain, or improvements in their movement. This awareness is part of the process. I won't deny that relearning how to move can be frustrating, especially if you moved better at some point in your life. It is natural to want to regain good movement *now*, rather than over months or even weeks, but understand that this takes time. Practice moving better each time you exercise, and be kind to yourself.

Guess what? The practice never stops. When you reach a point where you can confidently perform a squat without overthinking, you've hit a sweet spot. But that doesn't mean you stop there. Instead, find ways to make the movement a bit more challenging and start practicing again. That is how you continue to progress—step by step, rep by rep!

The Benefits of Repetition

It is no secret that repetition is key to improving any skill, and this is true across all forms of exercise. Whether you are dancing, lifting weights, gardening, or playing tennis, repetition offers significant benefits. It helps refine movements, build efficiency, and enables progression to the next level. With each repetition, there is always an opportunity to learn something new, whether through personal discovery or by learning from those who have mastered the skill.

Both the physical and cognitive benefits of repetition are vital. For instance, when a client improves their squat form, we can introduce additional weight, resistance, or new variations of the movement to increase the challenge. The more they repeat the movement, the more familiar their body becomes with it, resulting in decreased mental effort to perform it.

A story featured on NPR's *Fresh Air*, titled "To 'Keep Sharp' This Year, Keep Learning, Advises Neurosurgeon Sanjay Gupta,"[1] discusses the neurological advantages of learning and highlights the brain's capacity to generate new cells during the learning process. This underscores how learning new movement patterns through repetition not only benefits your body but also nurtures your brain.

Similarly, NPR's *Morning Edition* aired a segment titled "Learning A New Skill Works Best to Keep Your Brain Sharp,"[2] which discussed research indicating that acquiring new skills is crucial for maintaining brain function and health. The segment also referenced another study showing that "just 45 minutes of exercise three days a week . . . increased the volume of the brain even for people who have been very sedentary"[3] and helped resist memory loss. A neuroscientist involved in this study, "Exercise Training Increases Size of Hippocampus and Improves Memory,"[4] stated: "We found that exercise, even for people who haven't been exercisers and are very sedentary tends to improve a number of different aspects of cognition, including executive function, which includes things like planning, scheduling, multitasking and working memory."[5] These findings emphasize the value of moving more and learning to move better. Both your brain and body reap the rewards of consistent, thoughtful exercise.

The Pitfalls of Repetition

Although repetition is valuable, it has its limitations. For example, if you run five miles every day at the same pace and on the same route, your body will adapt, causing your progress to plateau. Without introducing new challenges—like adjusting your running time, incline, distance, or speed—your progress may stall. Varying even one aspect of your routine can help maintain a proactive and evolving approach to your health and fitness. Those who stick to the same workout day after day are more likely to miss out on seeing the results they are aiming for.

Moreover, continuously performing the same movements in the same fitness modality, such as running or cycling, can lead to tightness and reduced mobility if not balanced with stretching and mobility work. Runners who are tight can lose optimal running form and increase their risk of injury. For instance, during my half-marathon training, I overlooked stretching and mobility exercises. The resulting tightness affected my stride and made running uncomfortable. In everyday life, we rarely move in straight lines; our bodies are designed to move in multiple directions. Therefore, if you regularly cycle, run, or engage in other modes of exercise that mostly utilize the same movements, it is important to diversify your movement patterns to keep tightness and injury at bay and improve overall performance and functional capacity. Exercise does not have to happen solely in a gym or involve conventional workouts. Strength training or balance work can complement your hobbies, such as kayaking or golfing, and boost your confidence to tackle new challenges like hiking or travelling without worrying about your physical capability.

Be consistent with movement, but don't shy away from variety. Adding subtle variations to what you already do—such as adding weight to a squat or changing the tempo of a run—can make a big difference. The goal is to move better each day in ways that extend beyond your usual activities.

Striking the Right Balance

Everyone's "sweet spot" when it comes to exercise is different. It is common to ask a fitness professional or a successful friend, *What should I do?* But the truth is, whatever exercise routine you choose needs *your* buy-in. It should be something you enjoy or, at the very least, appreciate for the results it produces. If you dislike your chosen activity and don't see results, you are likely to lose motivation and give up.

A common misconception is that exercise must be grueling or something to suffer through—"no pain, no gain" or "if you're not crawling out of the gym, it wasn't a good workout." This mindset can lead to burnout and injury. Better movement may involve moments of discomfort but remember that discomfort is different from pain. Exercise, like any challenge, should push you in a way that helps you grow. There should be periods of ebb and flow— periods of easier effort (like practice tests) that prepare you for more challenging moments (like final exams). Exercise should provide opportunities to demonstrate what you and your body have learned so far. These challenges serve as reminders of your progress and highlight areas for improvement.

At times, you will need to push a little harder. If you do injure yourself, use it as a learning opportunity: reset, recover, and return with a better plan. If you experience soreness, remember that delayed-onset muscle soreness (DOMS) typically lasts about three days. If soreness lasts longer, adjust your approach and learn from that experience as well.

Practicing Better Movement Makes Daily Life Easier

Let's circle back to the squat that Don practices in the multiple-choice scenario earlier in this chapter. Since starting his sessions with you, Don has been doing squats along with other exercises. Over time, he has improved his confidence, balance, and ability to get up from a seated position without rocking. He has even progressed to holding a ten-pound medicine ball while standing up.

When Don is not with you, he carries out everyday life activities. The more he practices squats in his sessions and thinks about how to improve his form, the more these improvements carry over to his daily life. He notices he can get out of a chair at home more quickly, without needing to push off with his hands or rock. Even tasks like getting up from the toilet—a notoriously low seat—are easier now. He is excited about his newfound ability to move his body more efficiently and comfortably. Don's increased strength, stability, and confidence are due in no small part to the consistency and practice he puts into your sessions. This is why consistency, whether in sessions with a personal trainer or your own workouts, is key. Practice makes better!

Your Better is YOUR Better

Your better movement is better for *you*. Returning to Don—if you asked him to perform an Olympic lifter's squat, would that be his version of better? For many, this may be an impressive squat, but for Don, it would be a far reach to perform safely. His version of better is being able to get out of a chair without rocking and to perform a squat that minimizes pressure on his knees. His next step might be to do squats at a similar depth but without using a chair for support. Eventually, he could progress to holding external weight in his hands while squatting.

Don's body moves the way it moves, and there is no room for judgment or comparison. The goal is to help him move better *where he is today* and continue taking steps toward better movement. For example, if Don's squat form looks great but he experiences pain—or worse, increasing pain—that is not better. The goal is to help him move at the edge of pain, where the movement is safe and manageable for him.

It is important to understand the distinction between pain and discomfort. For example, discomfort for Don might include his legs shaking or feeling fatigued after completing twenty squats. He may find the movement difficult, feel out of breath, or experience soreness for the next day or two. Such soreness is often part of the process of getting stronger.

Your better is better for *your* body. Your body is unique, as is your life and your journey toward better movement. Don's history—whether it includes a long period of inactivity or years working in desk jobs—shapes his physical capabilities today. If Don had instead been a park ranger or a PE teacher, his physical history, strengths, and areas for improvement would look very different. The same goes for you. Your body has been with you through all the events in your life: injuries, sports, childbearing, raising kids, working at a desk, or even playing pickleball every weekend.

What matters most is that you start taking action now, being mindful of your current physical state. Wishing you had done something differently in the past will not change your circumstances today. And attempting to make up for lost time can be a recipe for disaster. Cramming for a test at school may work for some, but cramming doesn't work for fitness. Doubling up on reps, adding more weight than you should, or suddenly increasing the duration of your workouts are all risky choices that can lead to negative consequences. Similarly, going all out by jumping into an intense exercise schedule—like working out every day after a long hiatus—can also backfire. Start small. Exercise twice a week, then build up to three times a week. Incorporate other forms of movement into your daily routine, such as playing tennis, gardening, or even dancing. If getting back on the exercise train feels daunting, this might be a good time to invest in a fitness coach. A coach can help you create a program tailored to your needs, ensuring that you move better, stay consistent, and avoid injuries.

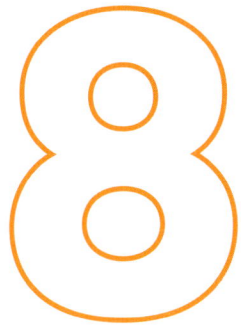

FALL PREVENTION 101

> *As you grow older, you learn that you don't have to prove yourself to anyone. You just have to be.*
>
> —SIDNEY POITIER, *THE MEASURE OF A MAN:
> A SPIRITUAL AUTOBIOGRAPHY*

If you believe you are at no risk of falling because your balance is good, consider this: What specific steps are you taking to reduce that risk? While strength training or general conditioning can help tangentially, truly lowering your chances of falling requires a focus on balance training and other preventive strategies. Improving your balance does not guarantee you will never fall, but it does mean that, when combined with a healthy diet that supports bone strength, you will have greater confidence, agility, and a lower likelihood of suffering a debilitating injury if a fall does occur.

Let's look at some statistics. According to a report from the Centers for Disease Control and Prevention (CDC), "Falls are the leading cause of fatal and nonfatal injuries among adults aged ≥65 years (older adults). During 2014, approximately 27,000 older adults died because of falls; 2.8 million were treated in emergency departments for fall-related injuries, and approximately

800,000 of these patients were subsequently hospitalized."[1] These numbers underscore how serious the consequences of falls can be—and why you need to take proactive steps to lower your risk.

You might know someone who has fallen. Perhaps you have experienced a fall yourself. Or maybe you think: *That won't happen to me.* It is time to stop assuming you will never be part of those statistics and start taking deliberate action to reduce your chances of falling.

A fall that leads to injury or hospitalization can be devastating—not just for your pocketbook but also for your mental health. The fear of falling again can creep in, especially if the incident occurred during a routine activity. This residual fear, influenced by the severity of the fall and the circumstances under which it happened, can spiral into a detrimental cycle of avoiding movement altogether. Falling inflicts more than physical bruises; it can also shake your confidence. In severe cases, individuals may avoid walking or even being on the floor. However, this avoidance increases the likelihood of future falls because when you stop moving with confidence and purpose, you weaken your ability to move safely.

Does aging automatically increase your risk of falling? No! Falls are not an inevitable part of growing older. They can happen to anyone at any age. Distractions, hazards in your surroundings, or even a moment of inattention can result in a fall. Take my experience as an example. Once, while trail running, I noticed two people walking toward each other on either side of the trail. I was focused on navigating around them and failed to notice a tree root in my path. The result? A spectacular fall. A client of mine once tripped over a concrete parking block while admiring Christmas tree lights. The lesson here is simple: Things happen, but it is crucial to learn from our falls and adjust our habits accordingly. After my accident, I made a conscious effort to watch for obstacles on the ground ahead. My client has also become more aware of her surroundings, likely pausing to admire decorations instead of continuing to walk while looking at them.

Imagine you are walking in an environment where you feel completely comfortable—your home, for instance. How would you walk? You would likely walk with a confident, natural stride, maintaining a wide and stable base of support. Now picture walking on a narrow, elevated walkway over a swamp teeming with your least favorite creatures. Chances are, your steps would become shorter, tenser, and more tentative—almost like walking on ice. You might even narrow your base of support due to your shorter strides. If you were to trip or need to move quickly, losing your balance wouldn't take much. This "tense walking" is problematic. The more you adopt a protective and hesitant way of moving, the greater your risk of falling becomes.

You may be wondering: *How can I reduce my chances of falling?* That's a great question. A solid fall prevention strategy involves multiple components. Let's discuss this in more detail.

Land-Based Exercises for Fall Prevention

Agility

An article on the American Council on Exercise (ACE) website defines agility as "the ability to move quickly and change direction with ease."[2] This definition applies to both physical and mental agility. Even if you are not a big sports fan, you have likely seen agility drills that football players and other athletes use—those quick footwork exercises designed to improve speed and the ability to change direction efficiently.

While you might not be training to become the oldest player in the NFL, incorporating agility training into your routine can enhance your confidence and body awareness. Gaining confidence in your ability to move your feet and body in different directions directly complements fall prevention.

Remember that anyone can fall, regardless of age. I took a tumble while trail running, not due to poor agility, but because I was not paying attention. Thankfully, I escaped with just minor cuts and scrapes. Some of my clients have also fallen without injury, but that isn't always the case. While agility training will not eliminate the possibility of falling, it will help you move better, react faster, and build the confidence to recover if you do stumble. When you lack confidence in your ability to move, you may tense up, hesitate, or avoid risky movements altogether, thus limiting yourself and creating a barrier to truly enjoying your life.

Here are some ideas for agility training:

- **Tennis ball drill.** Grab a tennis ball and throw it against a wall. Try to catch it before it bounces more than once. Challenge yourself to keep up with the ball, and have fun with it!

- **Weight shifting to balance.** Stand with your feet at least shoulder-width apart, distributing your weight evenly. Slowly shift your weight to one side, balancing on one leg while standing tall. Once balanced, return to the center, and repeat on the other side, reaching with the opposite foot, shifting your weight, and balancing. Repeat twelve times, but remember—quality beats quantity.

Balance

We rely on balance every time we are on our feet. It is only when balance starts to deteriorate that simple movements like standing up from a chair, walking up or down stairs, or reaching down to pick up something become difficult.

Improving balance involves much more than standing still on one leg, although that is a great starting point if that stance is challenging for you. In daily life, balance is dynamic. How often do you find yourself standing still on one leg during the course of your day? Rarely. Instead, you are often moving, twisting, or reaching. That is why balance training should mimic the dynamic nature of everyday movements. For example, you should feel confident walking up stairs, balancing on your tiptoes to reach for something high, or turning to grab something behind you—without worrying about losing your balance.

When my clients practice balance exercises, they are often multitasking. Why? Because balance is typically required while you are engaged in other tasks, like carrying groceries, cooking, or playing with grandchildren. For instance, my clients might perform bicep curls while standing in a position that challenges their balance or bounce a ball while shifting their weight. This way, they focus more on the task at hand rather than solely on balancing. While they may struggle to stay upright, balance becomes a secondary focus in the background. If multitasking feels like too much, you can always revert to focusing on static balance. There are many ways to tailor exercises to meet you where you are. The goal is to progress gradually. Once you are ready, challenge yourself to multitask or find other dynamic ways to train your balance instead of just standing on one foot waiting for time to pass.

Here are some ideas for balance training:

- **Tandem walk with head turn.** Begin by walking in tandem (heel to toe). Once that becomes easy, add a progression by turning your head left or right with each step, alternating sides. Walk slowly, focusing on rolling your entire foot from heel to toe as you move forward. Be mindful of your shoulders; don't let them rise up.

- **Single-leg balance with ball bounce.** Grab a tennis ball and stand tall on one leg. Once you are balanced, begin bouncing the ball and maintain your balance. Alternate hands to keep the exercise dynamic. To make it more challenging, lightly bounce the ball against a wall or play catch with a partner who is also balancing.

Stabilization

In their article, "Joint Mobility and Stability," ACE defines joint stabilization as "the ability to maintain or control joint movement or position . . . achieved by the coordinating actions of surrounding tissues and the neuromuscular system."[3] Think of this as staying in control. For example, if I asked you to step to the side in a variation of a lateral lunge, I would want you to fully own it—meaning, ideally, you would perform this movement with little to no wobbling. Variations of this lunge can be done while holding on to something for extra support if you need help stabilizing. When you move, it should be with strength and confidence, demonstrating your ability to hold a position with control.

Here are some ideas for stabilization training:

- **Half-kneeling Pallof press.** This is an excellent stabilization exercise, as shown earlier in chapter 6. Wrap a resistance band with handles around a sturdy pole or anchor point. Interweave one handle through the other to secure the band to the pole. Holding the free handle, step away to create moderate tension in the band. Turn so your right shoulder is in line with the anchor point. Kneel on your right knee, and place a pad under it for comfort if needed. Maintain a tall, upright posture. Interlace your fingers and hold the handle with both hands. Push the handle straight out in front of you, then rotate your torso to the left before returning to the starting position. Move with control and maintain balance throughout the exercise.

- **Slow squats.** Hold a light to moderately weighted ball or dumbbell in both hands. Lower yourself into a squat slowly while exhaling, simultaneously pushing your arms out in front of you until your elbows are locked. Move with control throughout the entire range of motion.

Strength

If you think you don't need strength to prevent falls, think again. One of the main body parts involved in fall prevention is—your legs. The strength to stand up, walk, climb stairs, or lower yourself into a seated position without plopping down all depends on maintaining strong leg muscles.

Here are some ideas for strength training:

- **Wall push-ups.** Face a wall and place your hands flat against it at shoulder height, with straight arms, palms up, and wrists aligned with your elbows. Your hands should be placed outside shoulder width, but if this feels uncomfortable, adjust by taking them wider. Lower your forearms against the wall while ensuring your posture remains upright. Walk your feet back a step or two so you are leaning slightly into the wall. Keep your knees locked and your hips elevated. Push away from the wall to straighten your arms, then lower yourself back until your forearms are on the wall again.

- **Weighted squats.** If air squats (bodyweight squats) are becoming too easy, it is time to add resistance. Hold a medicine ball or dumbbell close to your chest and perform a squat to your usual depth. Keep your form controlled, and avoid allowing momentum to take over as you move.

For both exercises, repeat the movements for a full set of ten to twelve reps.

Hearing and Vision: Key Components of Fall Prevention

Untreated hearing loss can affect far more than your ability to hear what is happening around you. A compelling article in *The New York Times* discusses findings from two studies that show "a clear association between untreated hearing loss and an increased risk of dementia, depression, falls and even cardiovascular diseases."[4] The article also mentions that for a significant number of people, the studies indicate that uncorrected hearing loss may actually cause associated health problems.

Research from Johns Hopkins found that:

People with a 25-decibel hearing loss, classified as mild, were nearly three times more likely to have a history of falling. Every additional 10 decibels of hearing loss increased the chances of falling by 1.4-fold. This finding still held true even when researchers accounted for other factors linked with falling, including age, sex, race, cardiovascular disease, and vestibular function. Even excluding participants with moderate to severe hearing loss from the analysis didn't change the results.[5]

The lead researcher of the study, Dr. Frank Lin, offers possible explanations for the link between hearing loss and falls. One reason is that reduced auditory input can lessen a person's awareness of their overall environment. Another reason is the cognitive load imposed by hearing loss, overwhelming the brain with demands on its limited resources. Dr. Lin explains: "Gait and balance are things most people take for granted, but they are actually very cognitively demanding. If hearing loss imposes a cognitive load, there may be fewer cognitive resources to help with maintaining balance and gait."[6]

What do these findings imply? Untreated hearing loss can raise your risk of falls. Although this may be an oversimplification of thorough and extensive research, the connection is clear: Our body is interconnected in ways we might not fully realize.

The relationship between visual impairment and the risk of falls is perhaps more intuitive. If you cannot see obstacles clearly, your likelihood of tripping or falling increases. Vision is also crucial for our ability to maintain balance. A study titled "Visual Risk Factors for Falls in Older People," published in the *Journal of the American Geriatrics Society*, highlights the link between vision and fall risk: "[A] loss of edge-contrast sensitivity may . . . predispose [older people] to tripping over obstacles within the home, and outdoor hazards such as steps, curbs, tree roots, and pavement cracks and misalignments."[7] Edge-contrast sensitivity refers to the ability to see the boundaries between objects, such as the edge of a step versus the ground or a raised surface between rooms. Older adults who struggle with this are more prone to trips and falls. These accidents are entirely preventable if visual impairments are addressed.

Depth perception is another key aspect of vision. If you wear glasses, you understand the importance of depth perception for navigating steps, curbs, and uneven surfaces. The same study indicates that: "Impaired depth perception was the best predictor of multiple falling. . . . Visual impairment, and in particular impaired depth perception, is an important risk factor for falls in older people."[8] When someone cannot accurately perceive how far down a step is or how high they need to lift their foot to clear an obstacle, their risk of tripping and falling increases.

So, how much of this visual loss can be corrected? Fortunately, the study suggests that much of the visual decline in older adults can often be remedied with simple interventions, such as a change of glasses or undergoing cataract surgery. In other words, being proactive about eye care—through regular eye exams and necessary corrective measures—along with removing tripping hazards from homes and public places, can significantly prevent falls and injuries.

Addressing vision and hearing impairments is an important aspect of fall prevention strategies besides training at the gym. These are simple yet impactful ways to improve your safety in daily life. Don't neglect regular checkups for your hearing and vision—your safety depends on it.

Fall Prevention: Water-Based Exercises

Fall prevention exercises can include working out in the water. If you have access to water aerobics classes or can exercise in a pool, take advantage of these opportunities. Moving and exercising in water is not only low-impact but also beneficial for the joints, especially when the water temperature is warmer. (Facilities offering Arthritis Foundation Water Aerobics classes typically maintain the water temperature between eighty-two and eighty-eight degrees Fahrenheit.) Don't confuse *low-impact* with easy! Like any land-based exercise, water workouts come with varying levels of difficulty. The classes you take may not require equipment, or they may use tools like water aerobics dumbbells, foam noodles, ankle cuffs with fins, or webbed gloves. Each of these items adds a different level of resistance when moving through the water. If swimming is not your strong suit, you can still participate in most classes as they are usually conducted at a water depth where you can stand.

Foot Health for Fall Prevention

Your feet are the foundation that gets you where you need to go, yet many people overlook their care and the mobility of their ankles. In my experience, individuals often focus primarily on their legs and above when it comes to exercise, mobility, or overall care. We tend to take for granted what our feet can do, even though they are the very base upon which we move. However, getting a foot massage can be an eye-opening experience.

When walking upstairs or up an incline, you should be able to raise your leg and flex your foot toward you as you climb, pushing off as you go forward. Shuffling or feeling as if your ankles are locked or stiff can negatively impact your gait, particularly in how you navigate obstacles, however small they may be. Conditions like bunions can affect your balance and lead to further complications.

The Framingham Foot Study, a cross-sectional study of older adults, shows a significant association between the severity of foot pain and falls.[9] The researchers noted the need for further research to examine how foot pain affects fall risk and potential interventions to reduce it. Nevertheless, it is easy to see how foot pain can affect movement. Walking gingerly or cautiously to avoid pain can increase the likelihood of falling. Pain can also make it harder to move quickly and confidently to avoid obstacles or regain balance.

The study also highlights that:

> While mild foot pain did not affect the odds of falling, moderate to severe foot pain was associated with increased odds of recurrent falls. This cross-sectional study also showed a significant relation between foot posture and falls in which participants with a planus foot [flatfoot] posture had an increased odds of recurrent falls compared to those with the normal foot posture. These results indicate that foot pain and foot posture may play an important role in recurrent falls among older adults.[10]

So, what is the main takeaway from this study? Many individuals may not realize that walking with pain or having flatfeet can lead to compensatory changes in posture, ultimately increasing the risk of falls. Even the best balance training regimen may be ineffective if foot pain is not addressed.

If you experience foot pain, consider what steps you are taking to address it. Do you stretch the bottoms of your feet by rolling them? Have you tried soaking them in Epsom salt baths after being on your feet all day? Have you changed the type of shoes you wear or ensured you are properly sized for footwear? Are you squeezing your feet into high heels? Shoes that are too tight will harm your feet. Many brands now offer a wider toe box to allow your toes to sit more naturally instead of being cramped.

Keep in mind that each foot contains twenty-six bones and a significant amount of connective tissue. Conditions like diabetes can affect your feet, circulation, and connective tissue. Consult a qualified professional to discuss your foot health and learn how to take care of them properly.

The flexibility and mobility of your feet and ankles can significantly affect how you move in daily life. Better care of these areas is easy to overlook when your focus is on improving balance or agility to reduce your chances of falling. Here are some ideas for taking care of your feet and ankles:

- **Rolling the bottom of your feet.** Use a tennis ball to apply gentle pressure while seated. Start at one spot, apply pressure for five seconds, then release and move to another point on your foot. If you hit a painful spot, stay there, focus on breathing, and then continue to a nearby point.

- **Ankle flexibility exercise.** While seated, wrap a towel around the ball of your foot, holding one end of the towel in each hand. Gently pull on the towel as you point and flex your foot.

  Tip: There is no specific time required for either of these stretches, but try doing them for five minutes each day. Always avoid pushing into pain, and remember to breathe. Focusing on your breath signals to your body that all is well and helps it relax. So any time you feel tension or discomfort, breathe.

- **Toe spacers.** Consider using toe spacers or toe separator socks to spread your toes and promote mobility, especially if you have your feet in shoes all day. You can wear these while reading, watching TV, or even walking around your home.

A Holistic Approach to Fall Prevention

Reducing your risk of falls and maintaining a low risk over time involves several factors. In an insightful interview on National Public Radio (NPR) about fall prevention, Dr. Elizabeth Eckstrom, a professor and chief of geriatrics at Oregon Health and Science University, summed it up well:

> It's not just your balance, or it's not just your vision, or it's not just one pill that you're taking. If somebody wants to reduce their risk of falls, they should really think about all of the various ways: making sure you're wearing the right shoes, using a walker if you need it, getting off those risky medications. It's really important to tend to all of those little details to get your fall risk as low as possible. I encourage people to just work on that really, really hard. It's worth the trouble.[11]

There are various angles from which to approach fall prevention. The most obvious is through balance training exercises. However, addressing often-overlooked issues related to your feet, eyes, and hearing, along with reviewing your medications and their side effects, is also vital as they can negatively affect your balance. Although it can be a lot to consider, being proactive about your health sets you up for success. Do as much as you can to move better and care for your health in ways that minimize your risk of falling.

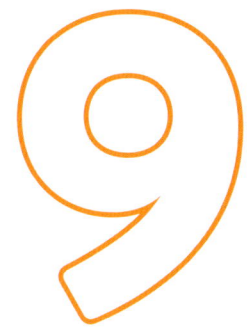

THE BRANCHES OF OUR PHYSICAL FUNCTION

> *Rather than viewing your body as a static biological machine . . . think of it as a field of energy and intelligence, constantly renewing itself.*
>
> —DEEPAK CHOPRA, *AGELESS BODY, TIMELESS MIND*

I want to delve into your physical function in a way that highlights how you can move better in everyday life and what the fitness professional working with you is (or should be) keeping in mind. On the next page is a valuable diagram, the Functional Aging Training Model (FATM), that was used in a certification workshop for the Functional Aging Institute (FAI). This organization focuses on educating personal trainers to help individuals aged fifty and older move better in life. This Functional Aging Specialist certification has been instrumental to my work with folks like you.

I will touch upon various aspects of physical function illustrated in this graphic. To save you from flipping back to this page as we progress through this chapter, I will zoom in on each specific section as we move along.

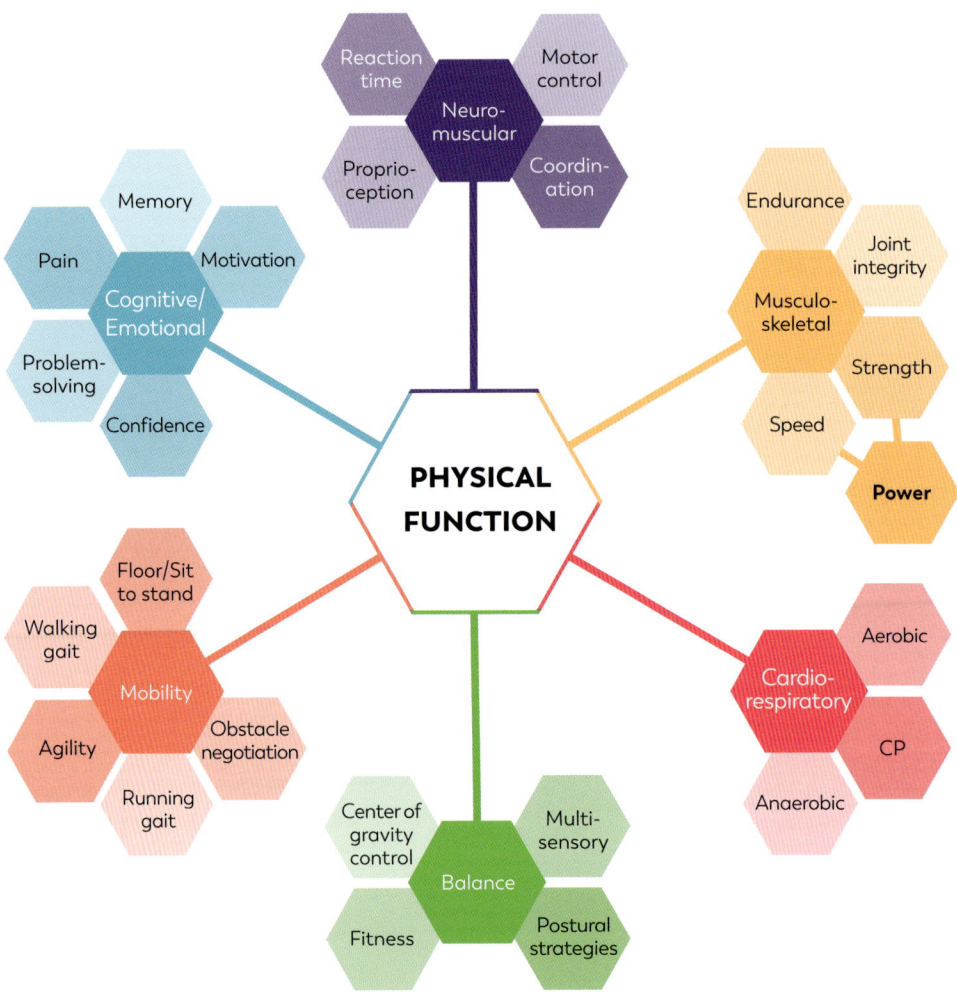

FIGURE 9.1. Six domains of physical function in the Functional Aging Training Model (FATM). Courtesy of Functional Aging Institute.

The Mobility Function

So, what exactly is mobility? Is it something I can find over the counter? Pete McCall, in his article "Stability vs. Mobility: What's the Difference?," describes joint mobility as a function that "relies upon a constantly changing axis of

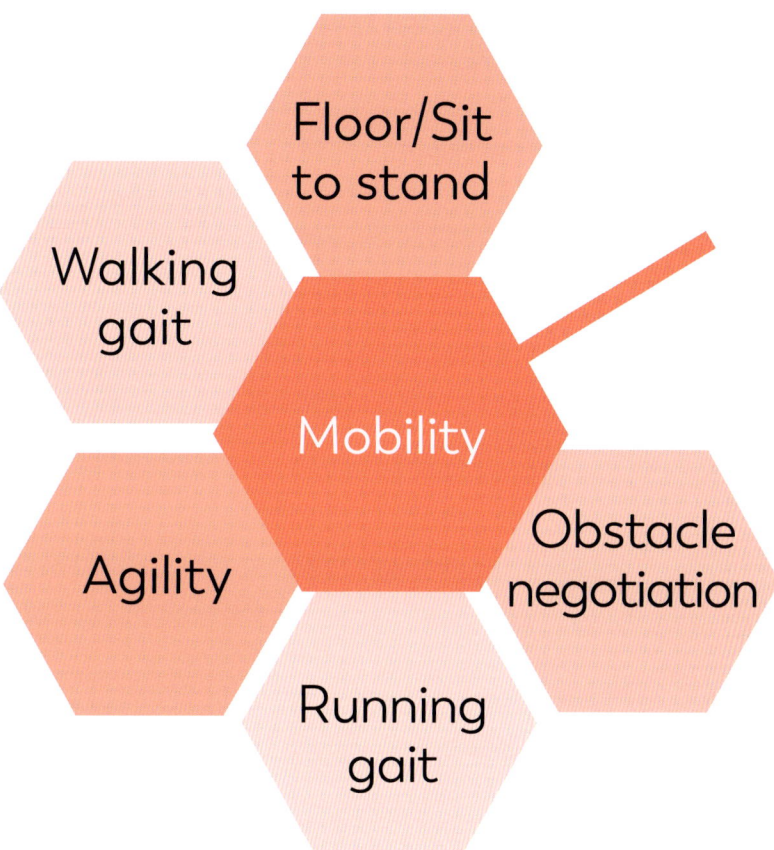

FIGURE 9.2. Mobility function, Functional Aging Training Model. Courtesy of Functional Aging Institute.

rotation." He further explains: "The muscle, fascia, and elastic connective tissue surrounding a joint function to create movement and provide the stability responsible for controlling joint position while it is in motion. Optimal mobility allows a joint to experience full, unrestricted motion while controlling the constantly moving axis of rotation."[1] Optimal mobility enables you to move your joints along a path and in a way that is natural and ideal for your body. This includes being able to raise both hands above your head or move your hips comfortably while walking, running, or moving without compensating for pain or discomfort. For instance, everyone's hips are unique, and so is their ability to squat at a certain depth. The placement of your feet can also affect how easily or deeply you can lower yourself. A position that works for me may not work for you. As mentioned earlier in this book, your body has a unique history that shapes how you move.

While the mobility you need to move around might not seem complex, it can feel overwhelming if you are experiencing a drastic decline in your range of motion. It can be daunting if you can't raise your hands high enough to place luggage in the overhead bin or retrieve something from a shelf. You may not even notice this decline because you have become accustomed to compensating, or alternatively, you might be acutely aware of your limitations.

Perhaps you think you can regain a full range of motion by pushing through the pain or forcing your body into a position you believe indicates full mobility. However, in reality, you are likely still compensating. Here is an activity you can try at home to illustrate this point:

1. Stand tall with your back against the wall.

2. Straighten one arm and make a thumbs-up with that hand.

3. Exhale and slowly raise your arm, aiming for your thumb to touch the wall.

The end point of your range of motion is just before you start compensating. Some signs of compensation include arching your back or flaring your rib cage.

What can help us maintain our range of motion? McCall explains, "Regular exercise and physical activity can ensure the elasticity of the attached connective tissues to provide functional performance when needed."[2] While this may sound simplistic, consistent exercise and physical activity are indeed essential for maintaining and improving your range of motion. The word to emphasize here is *regular*. Regular does not mean occasional. It doesn't mean only when you feel like it or just before a vacation to look good in photos. It means making a consistent effort over time. There are a variety of physical activities available to you regardless of your circumstances. Choose something you are interested in and start moving.

Hand in hand with regularity, it is important to stretch and move in different ways. I understand that these activities can feel boring, and it might seem like you don't have time for them. Still, you check off your designated workout for the day and move on. There is real value in any variation of movement that enhances mobility, and it does not have to include weights or equipment. Personally, I find that dynamic movement is more beneficial than static stretching, but you should do what works best for you. As I mentioned in chapter 5, a disclaimer for folks who are very flexible is to incorporate strength training to ensure you have the stability to own a position.

Taking the time to move provides rewards beyond improved mobility, such as better body awareness and a reconnection with where your body is in space. As you become more familiar with how your body moves, you may have some lightbulb moments, such as realizing that you are tighter on one side than the other (this is completely normal; we all tend to have a dominant side).

Lastly, let's talk about the word *functional* in McCall's quote. This term is often overused in the fitness industry, but McCall uses it for good reason. Mobility that allows us to perform everyday activities and tasks is *huge*! I am not referring to the ability to bend and twist like a yoga expert or gymnast. Rather, I am concerned with your ability to move with ease and body awareness.

TAKE NOTE OF HOW YOUR BODY FEELS

When you take up an activity like tennis or dancing, you often start to notice where your body feels tighter or looser. You might also identify areas and moments where you experience twinges of pain or soreness. Pay attention to these sensations—they provide an opportunity to learn, ask questions, or seek out ways to help you move better. (It could be as simple as looking up "tennis stretches" in a web browser!) For example, having the ability to execute a cleaner overhand serve can make a big difference in your game. Maybe your body is tight from the way you sit while driving, or perhaps your posture isn't great, which could be limiting your shoulder mobility. If you are experiencing pain, now is not the time to be a hero and push through it. Instead, find ways to stretch and work on your mobility without pushing into pain, staying at the edge of it. Do what feels good, ask questions, or do some research to discover what can help.

The Cognitive/Emotional Function

The cognitive/emotional aspect of physical function is an undercurrent in everything we do. Let's start at the bottom of this graphic and move counter-clockwise through this section, beginning with *confidence*.

I once worked with a woman who broke down in tears as she told me she no longer believed she could move the way she used to. Yet, she ultimately accomplished something she thought was impossible—she got down to the floor and back up again, unassisted. I am not a miracle worker, and we didn't spend a significant amount of time together before she achieved this. So, what changed? Because she hadn't been as active as she once was, she assumed the movement I asked her to perform would be a struggle. If anything, the real challenge for her wasn't the movement itself—it was the learning process. The movement came together within minutes. I believe what made the difference was her trust in me. Trust is essential. I worked to earn her trust, and thankfully, she offered it with little hesitation. She didn't tell herself she couldn't do it (or at least, she didn't say it out loud). She tried. It wasn't perfect, but with some guidance and adjustments, she improved—and before long, she nailed it. Was it flawless? No. But perfection was never the goal. What matters is this: *She did it.*

Because of the confidence she gained, she reached out to her old trainer, whom she hadn't spoken to in years, and scheduled an appointment. Writing this now still makes me emotional because that moment embodies why I do what I do. Her newfound confidence could help her regain the motivation to continue exercising and be consistent.

A lack of confidence can hold us back in any area of life. I know this firsthand; it is something I have experienced in both my professional and personal life. We are human, and we don't like to fail. But sometimes, we get in our own way. One way to build confidence is to get help from a qualified professional. It is common to feel uncertain or frustrated when trying to improve your quality of life through exercise. Even if you are only seeking brief guidance or reassurance, it can be comforting to know that you are on the right track and that any struggles you encounter are part of the process. Another way to boost your confidence is to focus on what you can do right now. Often, when we look at a goal, we lose sight of what we have already accomplished or what we are capable of in the moment.

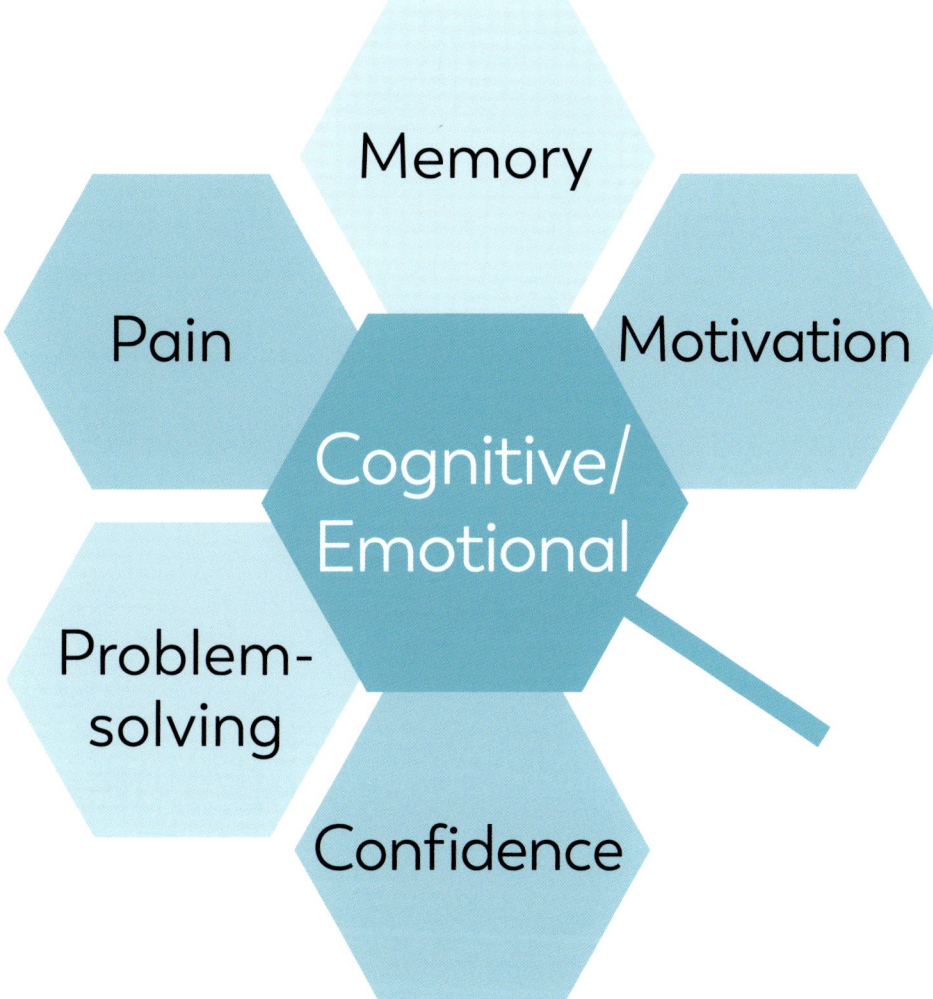

FIGURE 9.3. Cognitive/emotional function, Functional Aging Training Model. Courtesy of Functional Aging Institute.

Lastly, set yourself up for success. If you are acting as your own personal trainer, don't expect every workout to leave you exhausted or completely spent. Allow yourself time to practice better movement before introducing new, small challenges.

Let's look at the other "petals" around this section. *Problem-solving* is another crucial aspect. I like to introduce movements with clients that require them to think. Why? Because it taps into this problem-solving process. For instance, I might ask someone to balance on one leg and pick up a tennis ball in front of them. While this may sound simple, they must figure out how to balance while also lowering themselves in a controlled way to pick up something close to the ground—all without falling. The more they try, persevere, and eventually succeed, the more this benefits the emotional and cognitive aspects of their physical function. Remember, everyone progresses at their own pace toward "solving" the problem. Small wins are still wins, and setbacks happen to all of us. What's important is to keep on practicing!

Pain can indeed affect your emotions. It can make you avoid moving in certain ways. Even after the pain is gone, your body will remember it due to the neurological pathways that were created, causing you to continue moving in a protective or restricted manner. As discussed in earlier chapters, learning optimal movement techniques and engaging in regular structured physical activity can build strength and flexibility, helping to relieve pain and stiffness over time. This, in turn, boosts confidence and motivation to exercise consistently, creating a positive snowball effect.

Memory is a fundamental component of the cognitive/emotional function that we rely on throughout life. As mentioned in chapter 7, exercise and repetition positively impact memory and inhibit memory loss. In chapter 10, we will further explore how exercises that combine coordination and body awareness can enhance memory and brain function.

Motivation is a cognitive/emotional aspect that is closely linked to confidence in your ability to move with ease, as noted earlier in this section. Chapter 10 will also delve into strategies for boosting motivation (see "Fortitude: Exercising When You Don't Want to").

Neuromuscular and Cardiorespiratory Functions

You don't need to know all the ins and outs of the human body to appreciate how critical the neurological system is. Dr. Evan Osar and Jenice Mattek from the Integrative Movement Institute run workshops to educate fitness professionals on how to work with both the general population and special populations, such as active older adults. At one of their intensive two-and-a-half-day workshops, Jenice used a fantastic diagram and story to explain the central nervous system. Figure 9.6 is my re-creation of their diagram.

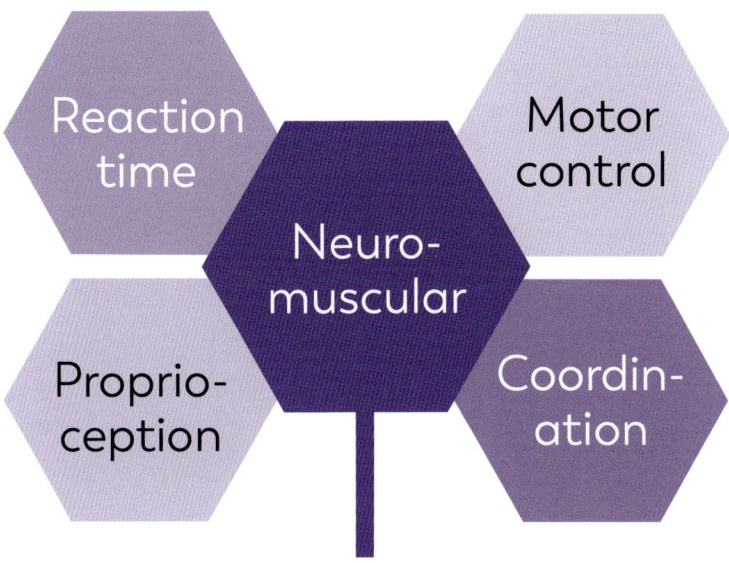

FIGURE 9.4. Neuromuscular function, Functional Aging Training Model. Courtesy of Functional Aging Institute.

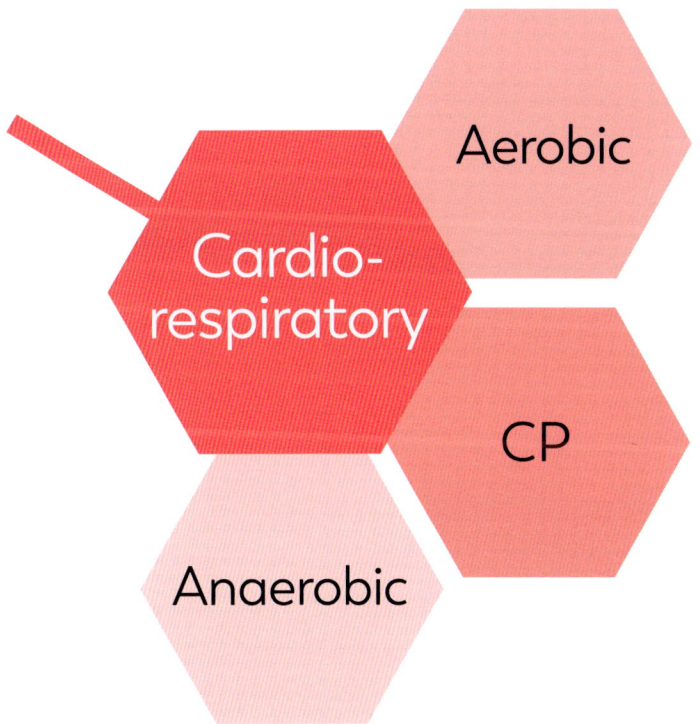

FIGURE 9.5. Cardiorespiratory function, Functional Aging Training Model. Courtesy of Functional Aging Institute.

The Central Nervous System —
The Role of Boundaries

1. Be home before dark.
2. Tell us who you will be with.
3. Stay within the boundaries
   we give you.

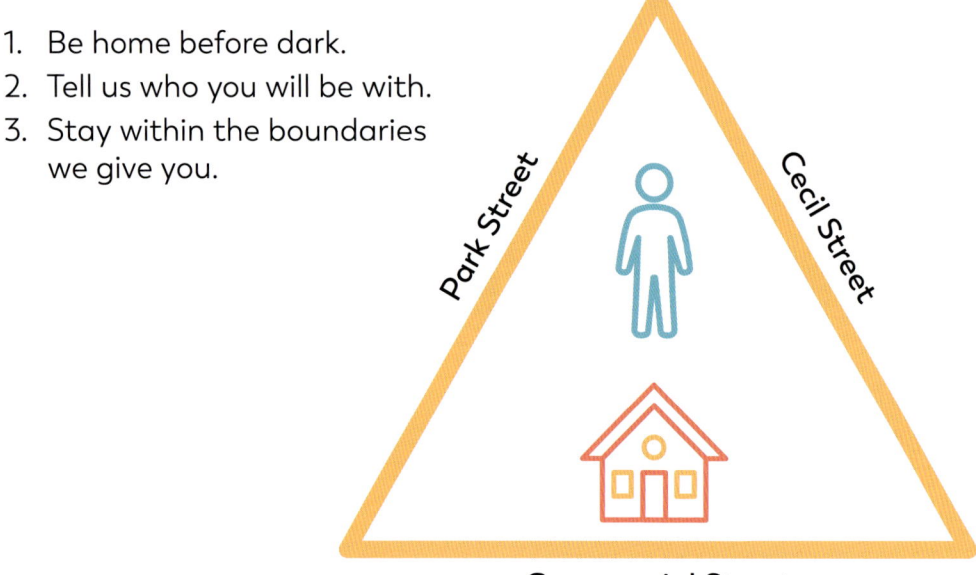

FIGURE 9.6. Adapted from an original illustration by the Integrative Movement Institute. © 2019, Integrative Movement Institute.

This diagram draws an analogy to the rules we follow as children. The three rules represent boundaries, while the three streets form the edges of the triangle. You and your house reside within this boundary. Let's take this a step further and discuss how these boundaries relate to the central nervous system.

Here are some key takeaways, paraphrased from the workshop with Jenice:

1. **Breaking the rules results in restriction.** If you venture outside the triangle (i.e., break the rules), you will face consequences, and your boundaries will be reduced.

2. **Restrictions require regaining trust.** If your boundaries decrease due to rule-breaking, you must earn the right (regain trust) to have your original boundaries reinstated.

3. **Maintaining trust leads to freedom.** If you consistently follow the rules, you will be rewarded with freedom within those boundaries. Over time, as trust is maintained, your boundaries can expand.

So, how does this apply to your body? If you adhere to the rules (or boundaries) of posture and movement, you will maintain your range of motion. This means you will retain and even gain the freedom to engage in the activities you enjoy. However, if you don't follow the rules—such as maintaining your body's most optimal alignment, breathing, and controlling your posture and movement—you will lose your range of motion. This loss often manifests as chronic tightness, discomfort, or increasing difficulty in performing everyday tasks and activities.

For instance, imagine you step outside your boundaries and attempt a deadlift with a weight that feels heavy to you. You know the proper form and alignment for a deadlift, but you are not ready for that particular weight and cannot execute the lift without compromising your form. But you do it anyway. While it may feel fine and even exhilarating in the moment, you could wake up the next morning with an aching back and a sore neck that hurts to move. Here's the key point: The deadlift itself wasn't the problem. The issue was ignoring the rules for proper form and alignment that would have protected your back while lifting that weight. You could have performed the exercise without experiencing painful aftereffects by using a lighter weight and sticking to the proper form. You essentially broke the rules and paid the price.

Now you must regain trust—whether that means undergoing physical rehabilitation or soaking in an Epsom salt bath. Either way, hopefully, you've learned your lesson. When you are ready to return to deadlifts, a smarter approach would be to gradually increase the weight in smaller increments while maintaining proper form and alignment.

By introducing challenges in a way that doesn't violate the rules, you will benefit from your training without risking injury. Strength training greatly benefits the neuromuscular system. As highlighted in the study "Strength and Endurance Training Prescription in Healthy and Frail Elderly," age-related declines in both neuromuscular and cardiovascular systems can be counteracted through exercise. Echoing my near-constant reminders of the importance of strength training, the study concludes that such training improves functional capacity, even for frail individuals who may think it is too late to begin. The researchers state: "Based on the current knowledge, it seems that exercise interventions that include endurance, strength, and muscle power training should be prescribed to frail elderly in order to improve the functional capacity."[3] In other words, if you think you are too weak or too old to start strength training, think again. It's never too late. Whether you are frail, strong, or somewhere in between, you can enjoy the benefits of a consistent strength training routine.

We previously discussed the significance of strength training for cardiorespiratory health in chapter 4 (under "Strength Train for Heart Health") and several effective cardio options in chapter 5 (under "Cardio and Options"). Refer back to those sections for a refresher on this crucial aspect of physical function.

The Musculoskeletal Function

Maintaining our musculoskeletal health is crucial, especially as we age. In *The Barbell Prescription*, the authors highlight the positive benefits of strength training on the musculoskeletal system. They explain: "Weight-bearing exercise improves bone density, joint function, tendon elasticity and strength, range of motion, and overall physical function."[4] This quote speaks directly to those of you who may worry about "getting big" or "too bulky" from strength training. Incorporating strength training into your routine is not just about building muscle; it is also about protecting your joints and bones. Does the word *osteoporosis* strike fear in you? If so, ask yourself: *What am I doing about it?* Both women and men need to incorporate some form of strength training into their lives. Set aside any assumptions that strength training is not for you due to your gender, age, or an existing injury. Strength is essential for navigating life. If you are unsure where to start, seek out a qualified trainer who understands your unique needs and can work with you, rather than relying on general advice.

Another key aspect to consider is *stability*, although it is not specifically mentioned in this diagram. I attended a workshop led by two leaders in the fitness industry, Tony Gentilcore and Dean Somerset, both of whom are renowned for their expertise in strength training. During their Hip and Shoulder Complex Workshop, they introduced the concept of *owning a movement*. Owning a movement is not just about being able to perform it; it is about executing it with control and confidence. It involves resisting weight or gravity without letting either dictate how you move. For example, doing a dumbbell press at a controlled pace is much more effective than simply throwing the weights up and letting them drop. Controlling the descent of the weight (deceleration) is just as important as pushing the weight up. In everyday life, owning a movement can mean squatting to gently lower a heavy or fragile

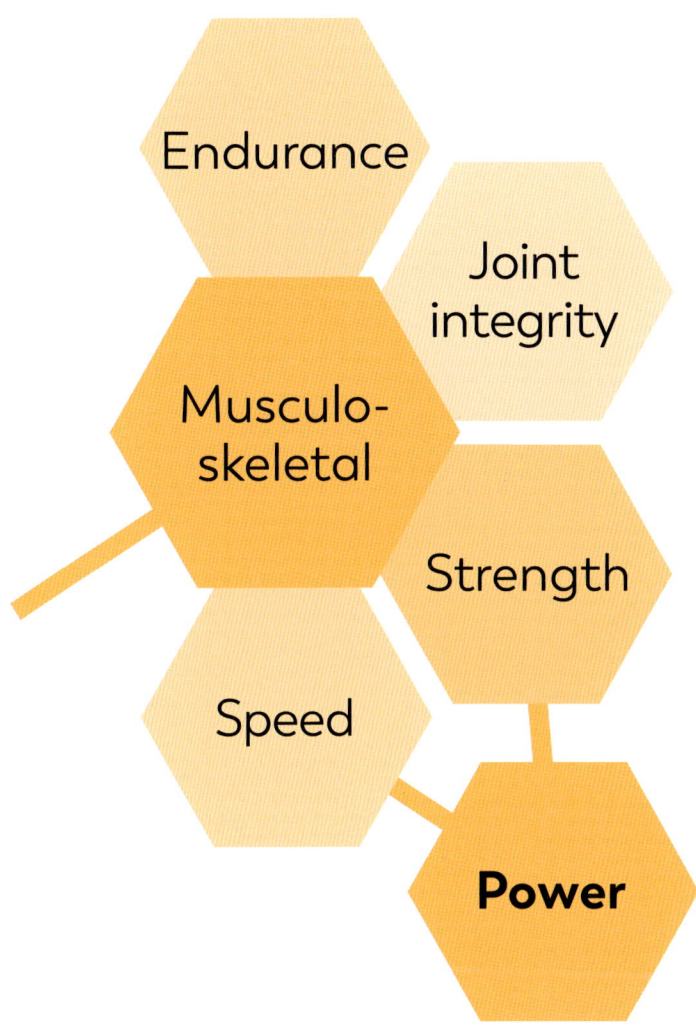

FIGURE 9.7. Musculoskeletal function, Functional Aging Training Model. Courtesy of Functional Aging Institute.

object to the ground. If you rely solely on gravity to do all the work, you risk breaking the object. Instead, owning the movement means lowering the object slowly and deliberately, with strength and control.

Balance

This diagram illustrates just how important balance is to our physical function. I dedicated a large part of chapters 4 and 5 to this topic, so I won't elaborate too much here. But I do want to emphasize again the critical need to

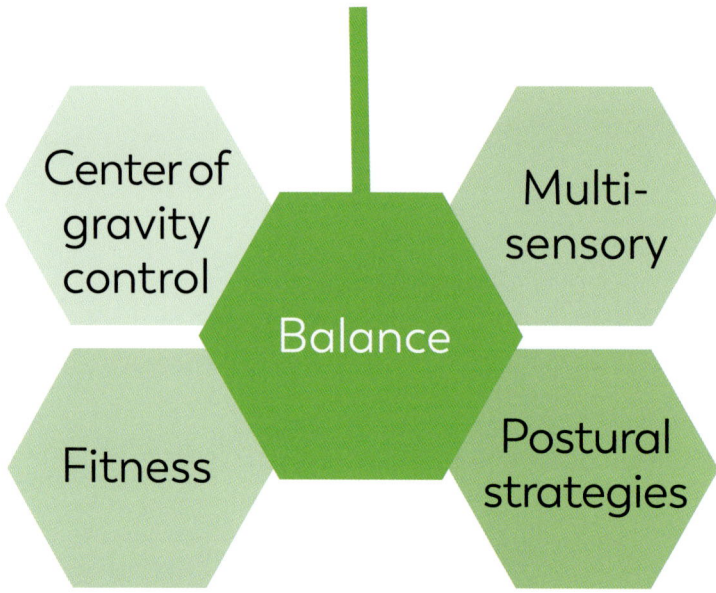

FIGURE 9.8. Balance function, Functional Aging Training Model. Courtesy of Functional Aging Institute.

start incorporating balance training into your routine if you haven't already done so. It doesn't matter how old you are, how good your balance is, or how poor you believe it to be—start practicing today. *Practice, practice, practice.* Begin where you are now and build from there.

✳ ✳ ✳

In this chapter, we have explored the key domains of physical function that affect how we move, balance, and navigate daily life. Each of these six elements of the Functional Aging Training Model is vital for maintaining independence and overall well-being. Understanding these interconnected systems empowers you to take proactive steps toward improving your movement quality, preventing injury, and boosting your confidence. The takeaway is simple: Movement and exercise are about maintaining your freedom to live life on your terms. Every effort you make to enhance your mobility, build strength, and work on your balance contributes to a stronger, more capable version of yourself.

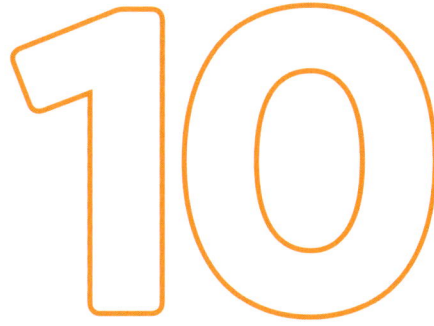

THE MENTAL ASPECT OF MOVEMENT

> *The human body is an incredible machine, but most people only get out of that machine what their mind allows them to.*
>
> —RICH FRONING, *FIRST: WHAT IT TAKES TO WIN*

Exercise is fundamentally a physical activity. But arguably, it is also heavily a mental act. Let's face it: Not all of us enjoy every single workout, exercise, or movement. Exercise demands physical effort as well as cognitive and neurological capabilities. No technology or magic pill can replace the effort required to exercise. You have to do it yourself. Simply having a gym membership is not enough. If it were, that secret would have gotten out by now!

Coordination, Body Awareness, and Memory

We need coordination in our everyday lives. The ability to move our hands, feet, and bodies in ways to complete tasks, engage in activities, and navigate our environment is an integral part of being human. When we are

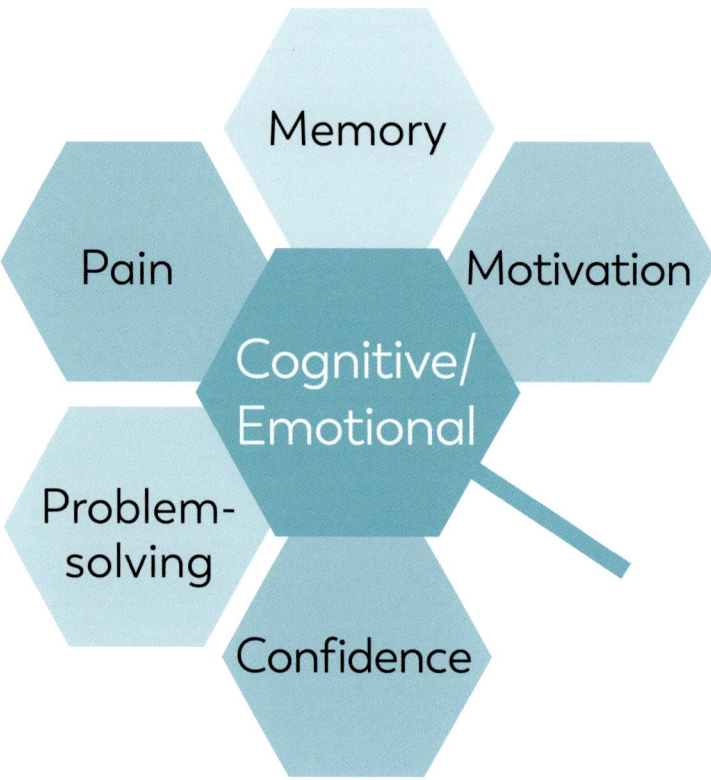

FIGURE 10.1. Cognitive/emotional function, Functional Aging Training Model. Courtesy of Functional Aging Institute.

active—however we define that—we rely on eye-hand coordination, dexterity, and agility. Remember the Functional Aging Training Model (FATM) we discussed in the previous chapter? The cognitive aspect of that model is closely connected to these abilities. While these capabilities may seem purely physical, they are significantly influenced by mental processes and have been shown to improve with exercise.

Dr. Cody Sipe, co-founder and VP of FAI, explains the cognitive benefits of exercise:

> [Exercise] tends to improve many aspects of cognitive function, particularly executive functioning, which is one of the most important. Executive functioning includes a wide array of cognitive processes such as attention, planning, problem solving, working memory, cognitive flexibility, abstract thinking, self-control, initiation of action, emotional regulation, inhibitory control, moral reasoning, and decision-making. Studies of the effects of exercise on cognition demonstrate more global improvements in cognition compared to cognitive interventions.[1]

The benefits of exercise extend well beyond building muscles or improving our appearance. When exercise is combined with coordination and other cognitive processes, it greatly enhances brain function. Our body and brain work in tandem seamlessly to handle countless tasks in the background while we move through life. The real work in exercise often lies in the cognitive aspect of performing a movement—remembering the steps to complete it and using coordination to execute them. For instance, in chapter 6 (figures 6.11 to 6.19), we observed Martha performing a floor-to-standing exercise known as the Turkish get-up. While I coached her through the steps, she had to physically move her body and remember where everything went. Clients often watch me demonstrate a movement, but when they try it themselves, they quickly realize it is not as simple as it appeared. This is where we break the movement down into steps, practice, and talk through the process. Over time, things begin to click, and they experience that rewarding lightbulb moment when practice pays off.

Isn't improved cognitive function an incredible benefit of exercise? As you can see, the body and mind are connected and synergistic when it comes to movement. Keeping this in mind, let's turn our attention to another vital aspect of cognitive function: body awareness.

Body awareness can be somewhat difficult to define, but it essentially refers to the ability to sense where your body is in space and to move it without needing to look or hesitate. For example, body awareness involves something as simple as rounding your back during a cat-camel or cow stretch or as complex as executing a Turkish get-up. Consider a practical example: You use body awareness when carrying a bag of groceries with both hands, navigating stairs, or stepping over obstacles without looking down. This awareness allows you to move and adjust based on verbal instructions, rather than requiring someone to physically guide or adjust you.

Incorporating exercises that utilize coordination and body awareness can make workouts far more stimulating. These exercises often require performing movements in specific steps, ensuring that certain limbs are moving while others remain stationary. When I introduce these types of exercises to my clients, I notice that their memory is challenged and their concentration levels go through the roof. They become fully engaged, even if they aren't as excited about the process as I am. I can see their wheels turning as they figure out how to manage the complexity. The reason clients may not find this process exciting is that there is often a lot to focus on at once. An exercise can be much more challenging in practice than it appears during a demonstration, as it is not only physically tiring but also mentally exhausting due to the concentration required and the need to remember the sequence of movements.

Nourishing Food for Your Noggin

Exercise offers numerous neurological benefits. I love telling my clients, especially when they are trying a new movement and feeling frustrated: *Your brain is loving this!*

A 2013 study titled "The Influence of Exercise on Cognitive Abilities" highlights the significant impact of exercise on the central nervous system. It discusses research in both humans and animals that supports the idea that exercise promotes cognitive health throughout our lifespan. The main focus of the study is the effect of exercise on the brain and cognitive abilities. The researchers conclude, "The evidence accumulated so far indicates that exercise is a strong promoter of cognitive health in humans."[2] While the conclusion continues with more specific language to support this point, that sentence alone is powerful enough. No need to get too caught up in details. What matters is understanding that cognitive health is vital, and as we age, its significance becomes even more evident. If there are ways to improve the health of our brain and central nervous system, we should pursue them actively.

The National Institute on Aging, part of the US Department of Health and Human Services, defines cognitive health as "the ability to think, learn, and remember clearly."[3] So let's connect the dots. Exercise improves your ability to learn, think, and remember—skills that are imperative for enjoying life and tackling routine tasks. This ability is central to living a fulfilling life. To reduce the likelihood of cognitive decline as much as possible, embrace exercise.

The study also looks back at our ancestors to shed light on the evolutionary link between physical activity and cognitive abilities:

> The active lifestyle of our early ancestors using locomotion and foraging may have demanded development of cognitive abilities for survival. The intrinsic ability of locomotion to engage energy transactions at the cellular level seems to have evolved simultaneously with molecular adaptations serving a cognitive function. In the modern age where industrialization has dramatically

transformed lifestyle, it is ever more so important to realize the dependency that the brain holds on physical activity and healthy dietary choices.[4]

Our lifestyles have changed dramatically since the days of hunter-gatherers. Today, there are more ways than ever to avoid moving our bodies. We no longer have to work physically for our food, and newer modes of transportation emerge each year, making it easier to get from point A to point B. Remote controls minimize physical effort, and elevators and escalators often allow us to skip stairs. In contrast, our ancestors' daily survival depended on physical activity. For them, every day was a struggle to find and collect resources—essentially, every day was a workout.

Fortitude: Exercising When You Don't Want to

No one wakes up every single day feeling completely excited to work out. That kind of enthusiasm only occurs on social media, in movies, or with people who aren't being entirely truthful! Life happens, emotions happen, and stress happens. However, the more you resist succumbing to excuses—whether it is to skip an exercise class, a strength training session, or a personal trainer appointment—the more you build a foundation for maintaining good habits.

But sometimes, life does get in the way. If you only have thirty minutes instead of your usual hour for exercise, make the best of it. I also struggle with wanting to stick to a perfectly planned workout schedule. But sometimes, it's okay to adjust and accept that you couldn't complete everything you planned to. It's just one day. If you want to hold yourself accountable, pour that remaining time and energy into your next session when you have more time. Permit yourself to be all right with shorter workouts when life intervenes. Instead of skipping exercise altogether or feeling frustrated, do what you can.

Your commitment to staying consistent is what will help you maintain or improve your quality of life. You can choose to take care of yourself now, starting at *your* good, instead of waiting until physical therapy is needed due to an avoidable fall or injury. Also, remember to resist the urge to compare yourself to how others move or exercise.

Often, people know they need to be more active but don't know where to start or who to turn to for help. Use this book as motivation to take that first step—whether it's walking into a gym, joining an exercise class, or speaking to a trainer who understands how to work with your unique challenges and needs. Start exploring your options:

- Set up a time to visit a gym and observe the environment. Note how the staff treats you and whether it feels like a good fit.
- Research the resources your city offers, such as free or low-cost community exercise classes.
- Look into local fitness meetup groups.
- Explore online fitness communities and virtual group classes.
- Consider hiring a personal trainer for virtual sessions.

Then commit to one or more of these options. Don't limit yourself.

Struggling to form an exercise habit? Here are some suggestions:

- **Start small.** Commit to one day a week for your workout and treat it like an appointment with yourself. This could be your time to go to the gym, take a challenging walk, or do a workout at home. Once you are consistent with this weekly appointment, add an additional day.
- **Prepare the night before.** Lay out your workout clothes and anything else you need, such as equipment or water, so there are no excuses to skip it because you "can't find your sneakers." If you usually eat before exercising, have your pre-workout snack ready to go.
- **Enlist a friend.** Having a workout buddy can help keep you accountable and motivated, making it less likely that you'll skip your workout. You won't want to let them down!
- **Get creative.** Use fitness apps to make exercise fun. I know a woman who competes with her daughter on a fitness app to see who can take more steps in a week. That sure is a fun and productive use of technology.

Above all, when you are ready to make a change and prioritize your health, remember: You don't have to set the foundation for your exercise habit alone.

Breaking the Cycle of Boredom

Some individuals get downright bored by exercise, especially when they repeat the same routine every time. Introducing variety into your workouts can help stave off boredom. A group class involving circuit training, for instance, can be highly effective. Circuit training involves moving quickly from one exercise to another, with each exercise done either for a set time or a specific number of repetitions. This format keeps things engaging and can be an excellent solution for those with short attention spans.

Boredom may also stem from the frustration of not seeing results yet. The reality is that achieving results takes time, and consistency is crucial during this waiting period. Ensure that your workouts are moving you toward your goals. One way to do this, for instance, is by incorporating adequately challenging weights during strength training. Even when you aren't seeing visible results, remember that you are still making progress. By moving better and more than usual—even just a couple of times a week— you are improving your movement patterns, building strength, and maintaining your health.

For those who feel bored and frustrated when results don't come quickly, this section may already feel annoying. But consider this: Do you find getting up from a chair boring? Is being able to pick up groceries and put them away boring? Or is having the capacity to go for a walk boring? These movements and abilities are anything but boring because they are a vital part of life. The alternative—losing the ability to perform these basic movements—leads to stagnation, chronic disease, and a lower quality of life, which I am sure you want to avoid. Find activities you enjoy that get your body moving, and then keep doing them.

Lastly, don't overlook foundational movements. These include squats, lunges, pulling, pushing, and twisting—essential movements we perform in everyday life. If you only want to do the fun things that avoid these foundational exercises, I would raise the caution sign. Consistency in practicing and improving these movements is critical for building strength and keeping the muscles around your joints strong. For example, if you enjoy playing sports like tennis, remember that relying solely on that isn't enough to meet all your fitness needs.

Is Something Else Holding You Back?

Perhaps you have encountered this advice before, or you already know the benefits of exercise but still struggle to commit. Is it possible something deeper is holding you back? It could be a lack of interest in exercise due to chronic disease, frustration from not seeing benefits, or a combination of both. You might be fixated on the past, focusing on what you used to be able to do, or you may be dealing with a condition that makes everyday movement exhausting or painful. This takes a huge mental toll.

If you identify with one or more of these challenges, pause for a moment and reassess. It may be time to seek out other forms of movement that tap into the mind-body connection. Consider practices like tai chi, the Feldenkrais Method®, yoga, Watsu aquatic massage therapy, or others. These approaches can provide a much-needed reset, helping you breathe better, release pent-up tension, and open up that "pressure valve" so you can reengage with exercise and movement.

Develop a positive association with exercise. Sometimes, we need a *reset* to develop a better relationship with exercise and movement. This reset could be as simple as getting a massage every few weeks to loosen tight areas and help you feel refreshed, ready to continue your fitness journey. A massage can also provide new insights about your body. A skilled massage therapist can point out areas of tightness, giving you an opportunity to listen, learn, and ask questions. The more you understand your body, how it moves, and what it needs, the better equipped you will be to care for it.

Mindset plays a significant role. Over the years, I have crossed paths with people who feel hopeless about their ability to move better. They often lament what they used to be able to do and struggle to envision a future where they can regain even a fraction of that ability. Instead of focusing on what you *used to do*, shift your mindset to what you *can do right now*. Be open to the idea that small steps can lead to better movement over time. Hopelessness can easily become a self-fulfilling prophecy if you let it take root.

Even when you are presented with all the facts about the mental and physical benefits of exercise, it is easy to hit a barrier. Don't let that elephant in the room—whether it is fear, frustration, or doubt—make you feel hopeless and stuck. Seek out help. Start with small, achievable movements. If you choose to work with a movement specialist, remember that progress requires your presence and effort. You need to meet them halfway. Celebrate the small wins—these add up over time.

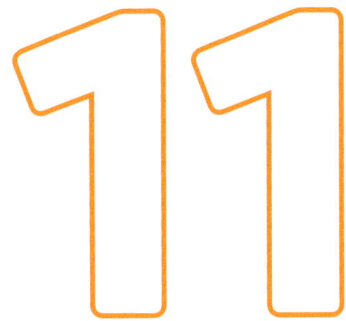

IT'S OKAY TO HAVE DESSERT

> *You can't help getting older, but you don't have to get old.*
>
> —GEORGE BURNS, *GEORGE BURNS: AN AMERICAN LIFE*

Wait. Don't just look at the title and think I am giving you carte blanche to drop the book and grab a generous slice of chocolate cake right now. But in a way, I am.

Curious? Here's the backstory: A client of mine occasionally experienced back pain when I first started working with her. She decided to stop sitting on the couch as much because she noticed her back would hurt after spending time on it, even though she is very active in her everyday life.

She later told me how happy she was to be able to watch the entire World Series without any back pain from sitting. Then, she tried to qualify her joy by saying she knew that sitting down is "bad" for her. I told her not to feel guilty about sitting down—it was her little treat, or dessert. There are activities and things we enjoy that may not be the best for us if they become habits, like sitting for long periods or indulging in sugary or calorie-heavy foods. But here's the deal: It is okay to enjoy dessert on occasion, especially when you have established good habits that enhance your quality of life. The reason her back pain diminished was that she showed up for our sessions every week and worked hard to improve her strength from head to toe. Her sessions were challenging, and at times, she felt frustrated—whether it was because of a bad day, not having eaten enough breakfast, or me throwing her a curveball by introducing a tougher movement. And that's okay—that frustration is natural. As exercises become more challenging, frustration can often be part of the process. The key is dedication and the commitment to showing up ready to work. Improvement comes with consistency.

Another factor in her reduced back pain was that she took initiative outside of our sessions. After consulting with me for suggestions, she committed to doing exercises on her own at home. She gets 100% of the credit for taking that step. She also stayed physically active in various ways beyond our sessions and her home workouts. Thanks to her tenacity, her back and core became stronger. She developed better posture when sitting and, perhaps most importantly, she learned to listen to her body.

Moderation is the key—both literally and figuratively—when it comes to dessert. Self-care habits and exercise are critical, but I don't want you to think you need to cut out dessert entirely. For example, another client recently told me she would be away for over a month to visit friends and take a road trip. She apologized for being gone so long. My response? I told her to enjoy her life. I would rather she live her best active life than be unable to physically do the things she loves.

Remember, having dessert every day is not a great idea, but enjoying a little now and then is perfectly fine. Move for life. Train for the life you want to live. And sprinkle in some dessert, just like adding salt to flavor a dish—just enough, not too much.

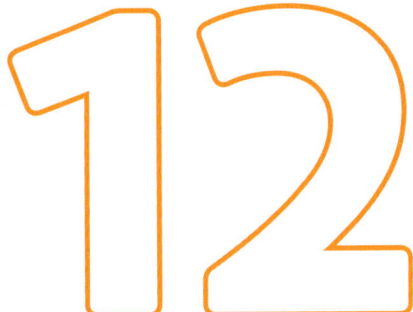

MOVE
FOR LIFE

> *People are surprised and tell me that I don't look my age ... but what is my age supposed to look like?*
>
> – MARTHA, A CLIENT

The three words that make up the title of this book encapsulate its essence. *Move for life* means to *move better for the life you want to live*. It means training to nurture both your body and mind so you can live a full and fulfilling life. It represents a mindset that rejects the notion that your best years are behind you and defies ageist ideas about what you should or shouldn't do because of your age. In a sense, this title is more than a theme—it is a conclusion. *We are all made to move.* This truth applies at every age and stage of life, even if we don't realize the importance of movement until we grow older.

This title does not refer to the life that society expects you to live or the one you feel pressured to live. It is *your* choice to define the quality of life you desire. You don't need to be a marathoner with a closet full of race shirts and medals, nor do you have to be an adrenaline junkie climbing mountains or skydiving. But you do need to be able to physically handle what life demands of you: the activities of everyday living.

If you are happy with your current quality of life, what steps are you taking to sustain it? Positive thinking alone will not maintain your quality of life. If you love how you feel now, start taking preventative measures today to continue feeling this way for as long as possible.

If you are not happy with your quality of life, what will you do about it? Don't fall into the trap of believing that nothing can be done and that things will inevitably fall apart. You can make small, positive changes to enhance your quality of life. These changes don't have to happen all at once. In fact, trying to overhaul everything at once—changing your diet, how much you exercise, or more—can lead to burnout. My advice is to take measurable steps and set attainable milestones instead of attempting to transform everything all at once.

Exercise is for everyone. In the study "Physical Exercise as a Preventive or Disease-Modifying Treatment of Dementia and Brain Aging," researchers delved into the cognitive benefits of exercise for older adults. While the focus was on reducing the risk of dementia, they presented a compelling statement about the broader benefits of exercise. The study noted:

> Numerous noncognitive, nonvascular benefits additionally benefit from exercise, which may be especially relevant to an aging population. This includes reduction of osteoporosis and fracture risk, age-related sarcopenia, and benefits directed at depression and anxiety. An exercise program may improve behavioral management in seniors with dementia and fall risk. Importantly, long-term physical activity and fitness reduce mortality risk in the general population."[1]

As you can see, this study highlights the substantial advantages of exercise for older adults. When you commit to exercises that build strength, improve balance, or enhance coordination and agility, you help mitigate the risks mentioned. You already perform squats every day when sitting and standing, and you likely lift objects weighing over five pounds several times in a day. These movements don't require gym membership, but neglecting regular strength and balance training could lead to losing these abilities over time. Making excuses like "I don't want to get too bulky or too muscular" can end up causing you to play catch-up later. Living your best life means maintaining the physical capability to do what you want to do.

Accept your story. If your story is that you sacrificed your health for your career, own it. Building your career took time, and it will take time to improve your quality of life to the level you believe you deserve. If you are dealing with chronic pain or tightness built up over the years, the solution could be as straightforward—or as challenging—as learning to breathe better. Whatever your story and goals may be, remember that *practice makes better.*

I believe in you. You have the potential to move better now so you can move even better tomorrow.

Thank you for taking the time to read my book. I wish you the very best on your journey to moving better in life. Feel free to reach out—I'm here to help you on that journey.

RESOURCES

This book focuses on better movement, but as an active ager, there are many other important aspects of life to consider. To address these, I've compiled a comprehensive list of resources spanning various facets of aging.

The resources include ones specific to San Diego for local residents, as well as online options for individuals outside of Southern California. At the time of publication, these resources are current. However, this is just the tip of the iceberg—countless additional tools and organizations are available for you to discover. I encourage you to do some sleuthing on your own as well! Many of the organizations and advocates listed here work in multiple aspects of exercise, wellness, and healthy living.

If you are reading a printed version of this book, you can visit www.move forlifebook.com to access all of these links in one place, saving you the effort of typing each URL yourself. Additionally, be sure to explore your local government and area-specific organizations for further support. This list is by no means exhaustive, but it's a great starting point!

INCREMENTAL FITNESS RESOURCES

On the Incremental Fitness™ website (www.incrementalfit.com), you'll find an ever-growing collection of videos and blog posts covering a wide range of topics.

SAN DIEGO-SPECIFIC RESOURCES

211 San Diego – Resources for Older Adults

This page provides access to a wide variety of agencies and resources for older adults, covering housing, legal services, and more.

www.211sandiego.org/olderadults

Aging & Independence Services – San Diego County

This county-run website lists a broad range of services for older adults, people with disabilities, and their family members. Available resources include mental health support, employment training, and much more.

www.sandiegocounty.gov/content/sdc/hhsa/programs/ais.html

Alzheimer's Foundation – San Diego

This foundation, which is independent of the national chapter, offers free services to support individuals with Alzheimer's and their caregivers. Resources include access to clinical care coaches, online education, and support groups.

www.alzsd.org

Feeling Fit Club

For those lucky enough to live in sunny San Diego, the county offers free fitness classes for older adults at various locations. Recorded classes are available online to follow along from the comfort of your own home, for those unable to attend in person.

www.sandiegocounty.gov/content/sdc/hhsa/programs/ais/health _promotions.html

Live Well San Diego

This partnership brings together businesses, health care providers, and community advocates to help San Diego residents of all walks of life and ages improve their health and thrive. The website includes an event calendar of wellness activities and community events, as well as resources on health-related topics across the country.

www.livewellsd.org

Oasis

Oasis offers a wide variety of classes, including instructional how-to sessions, educational courses, fitness programs, and many other resources, available both in person and online. A client of mine even took a course using her iPhone! Oasis has something for everyone.

https://san-diego.oasisnet.org

Sharp HealthCare – Senior Resources

Sharp Healthcare is a health care system in San Diego with hospitals, affiliated medical groups, and a health plan. It provides services such as health screenings, seminars, and other services and resources tailored for older adults.

www.sharp.com/services/seniors

Stein Institute for Research on Aging – UCSD TV

UCSD's TV department offers videos, links, and resources on topics related to healthy aging, such as plant-based sources of Omega-3s, nutrition, and diets for longevity.

www.ucsd.tv/stein

Stein Institute for Research on Aging – Public Lectures

The Stein Institute hosts free public lectures by renowned researchers and clinicians on topics such as sleep and how it impacts aging, effective Alzheimer's treatments, and other subjects focused on mental and physical well-being for active agers. Past recorded lectures are also available for viewing.

https://healthyaging.ucsd.edu/events/public-lectures.html

FINDING A FITNESS COACH ONLINE

Word of mouth is often a great way to find a fitness coach. If you haven't had luck with referrals, here are some online resources to help you locate certified fitness professionals.

American Council on Exercise (ACE)

ACE is a leading organization that offers general personal training certifications as well as specialized programs for fitness professionals. They also share helpful articles and videos for both fitness trainers and the general public. Their database provides a search feature to help you find ACE-certified fitness professionals in your area.

www.acefitness.org/resources/everyone/find-ace-pro

Functional Aging Institute (FAI)

FAI specializes in preparing fitness professionals to improve the quality of life for active agers. Through their certifications and workshops, they equip trainers to address the unique needs of older adults. Their searchable database can help you find an FAI-certified fitness professional near you.

www.functionalaginginstitute.com/find-a-fai-professional

Integrative Movement Institute (IMI)

IMI provides fitness professionals with various tools, including certifications, workshops, books, and free resources, to teach clients from all walks of life how to move better. You can use their database to locate a Certified Integrative Movement Specialist in your area.

www.discoverimi.com/imscertified

Original Strength (OS)

OS shares a unique and effective approach to movement that helps reset body functions like breathing and the central nervous system. The OS method also helps individuals connect with their bodies through movement, often in ways they have not experienced before. OS courses and certifications are open to both fitness professionals and the general public. Their website includes a database of OS-certified coaches.

www.originalstrength.net/find-a-certified-professional

EXERCISE DATABASES & TIPS

ACE Fitness – Exercise Library

This extensive and regularly updated library from ACE features exercises for all fitness levels. Each entry includes detailed instructions and helpful suggestions to ensure effectiveness.

www.acefitness.org/resources/everyone/exercise-library

HASFit – Exercise Library for Seniors

HASFit offers a variety of workout routines designed for older populations, ranging from beginner to advanced levels and with options of different lengths.

www.hasfit.com/workouts/seniors

Girls Gone Strong (GGS)

GGS provides advocacy and a supportive space for women looking to improve the quality of their lives through exercise, nutrition, and lifestyle changes. They also offer certifications and resources for fitness professionals who work with women.

www.girlsgonestrong.com

Movement Reborn – YouTube Channel

Based in San Diego, Andy Hsieh shares his knowledge on better movement techniques through informative videos for the general public.

www.youtube.com/c/movementreborn

Original Strength Videos

OS also offers a video library focusing on bodyweight movements to enhance mobility and flexibility. Their techniques are movement-based rather than static stretches and often incorporate breathing reminders to help "turn off" muscle tightness.

www.originalstrength.net/videos

SilverSneakers

SilverSneakers is a well-known advocate for fitness and wellness among older adults. Their program offers free live classes and workshops for those aged sixty-five and above with eligible Medicare plans.

https://tools.silversneakers.com

YMCA – Healthy at Home for Active Older Adults

The YMCA offers virtual, at-home workout programs for older adults, including yoga and tai chi, designed to keep you active and engaged.

www.ymca.org/what-we-do/healthy-living/at-home/active-older-adults

US NATIONAL ORGANIZATIONS

This section includes US national organizations categorized into the following areas: aging, caregiving, government, health, home safety, legal, LGBTQ+, travel and recreation, and special populations. Many of these organizations collaborate and overlap since they offer a wide range of services and resources, so be sure to explore them fully to see everything they can offer you.

AGING

American Association of Retired Persons (AARP)

AARP is a national organization focused on the interests, needs, and vitality of individuals aged fifty and up. Their website features articles on topics ranging from politics and society to scam and fraud prevention. They also provide resources to help individuals make informed decisions. Membership grants access to additional content and services.

www.aarp.org

American Geriatric Society (AGS)

AGS is a national nonprofit for geriatrics health care professionals, dedicated to improving the quality of life and independence of older adults. Their programs include initiatives for better care of older adults, such as those hospitalized with hip fractures. The site also features publications and resources for health care professionals who are AGS members.

www.americangeriatrics.org

Columbia Aging Center

Part of the Columbia University Mailman School of Public Health, New York, this center focuses on interdisciplinary research and education aimed at increasing healthy lifespans, creating well-being in our second half of life, and making longevity an asset. Peruse their website for content including globally focused research. Check out their seminar series to sign up for upcoming webinars led by experts in the field.

www.publichealth.columbia.edu/research/centers/robert-n-butler-columbia -aging-center

Gerontological Society of America (GSA)

GSA is the oldest and largest interdisciplinary organization devoted to research, education, practice, and public awareness in the field of aging. Their website features a vast catalog of on demand webinars on aging research, health management toolkits, and several other resources like the *GSA on Aging* podcast and the *GSA Momentum Discussions* podcast, which include interviews and conversations with leading experts.

www.geron.org/Resources

Leadership Council of Aging Organizations (LCAO)

LCAO is a coalition of nonprofit organizations advocating for policies that support the health and well-being of older adults in America. Their site provides information about their core issue areas, such as health, income security, and community services, along with current news and actions.

www.lcao.org

USAging

USAging is the national association representing the network of Area Agencies on Aging and Title VI Native American Aging Programs in Washington, D.C. They advocate for the needs of older adults through a range of programs and resources.

www.usaging.org

National Council on Aging (NCOA)

The NCOA provides advocacy for individuals aged sixty and older, as well as for caregivers and professionals. Their resources cover topics such as fall prevention, economic well-being, senior centers, and healthy aging programs. They partner with various organizations that prioritize the health and economic security of older adults.

www.ncoa.org

CAREGIVING

Family Caregiving Alliance (FCA)

FCA works to improve the quality of life for family caregivers and those receiving care. Their efforts include publications about caregiving issues and health conditions, as well as operating the National Center on Caregiving, which focuses on legislative advocacy.

www.caregiver.org

National Alliance for Caregiving (NAC)

NAC advocates for family caregivers and their care recipients through research, federal and state advocacy, and collaborations with like-minded organizations.

www.caregiving.org

National Association for Home Care & Hospice (NAHC)

This nonprofit represents home care and hospice organizations across the country, advocating for both the organizations and their employees.

www.nahc.org

SCAN Foundation

The SCAN Foundation is an independent public charity that aims to improve care and supportive services for older adults while emphasizing their independence.

www.thescanfoundation.org

GOVERNMENT

Administration on Aging (AOA)

The AOA is the principal agency of the US Department of Health and Human Services, tasked with carrying out the provisions of the Older Americans Act of 1965. It oversees numerous programs that provide resources to the public on topics such as brain health, oral health, and HIV/AIDS.

www.acl.gov/about-acl/administration-aging

US Department of Health and Human Services (HHS)

The HHS works to improve the health and well-being of all Americans by offering a broad range of services and resources, including caregiver support programs, public health and safety initiatives, and explanation of rights under HIPAA regulations.

www.hhs.gov

Medicare.gov

This is the official website for Medicare. Here, you can access information about your plans and find resources related to available coverage options.

www.medicare.gov

National Institute on Aging (NIA)

The NIA conducts research to understand the nature of aging and to extend the healthy, active years of life. It also provides health information informed by research and reviewed by experts to help the general public learn about healthy aging and common health conditions in older people.

www.nia.nih.gov

US Department of Veterans Affairs (VA)

The VA's mission is to serve veterans benefits and maintaining a nationwide health care network. Its services address the unique needs of minority and homeless veterans, among others.

www.va.gov

US Department of Agriculture (USDA) – Older Individuals Resources

The USDA provides resources tailored to seniors, covering a range of topics such as nutrition and healthy eating, as well as food security assistance programs.

www.nal.usda.gov/fnic/older-individuals

HEALTH

American Heart Association (AHA)

The AHA offers information and resources to help individuals build and maintain a healthy lifestyle. Topics include sleep, healthy eating, stress management, and recognizing heart attack and stroke symptoms. Professionals can also find resources like workplace health programs and CPR course registration.

www.heart.org

Arthritis Foundation

The Arthritis Foundation advances and shares the latest research on arthritis and offers valuable tools and information for disease management.

www.arthritis.org

The American Association for Geriatric Psychiatry (AAGP)

This organization focuses exclusively on geriatric psychiatry and the mental health and well-being of older adults.

www.aagponline.org

Meals on Wheels America

Meals on Wheels delivers nutritious meals to older adults while also engaging in advocacy and conducting research on topics like food safety and in-home safety issues for the older population.

www.mealsonwheelsamerica.org

Medicare Rights Center

This nonprofit provides counseling, advocacy, educational programs, and public policy initiatives with the goal of affordable health care for older adults. It also assists individuals in navigating the complexities of the Medicare system.

www.medicarerights.org

National PACE Association (NPA)

NPA supports Programs of All-Inclusive Care for the Elderly (PACE), a program that allows older adults who need nursing home care to continue living in their homes and maintain their independence for as long as possible, while receiving comprehensive health care. Its efforts include working with policymakers and collaborating with like-minded organizations in Washington, D.C.

www.npaonline.org

HOME SAFETY

National Directory of Home Modification and Repair Resources

This nationwide directory is provided by the Fall Prevention Center of Excellence, a project of the University of Southern California Leonard Davis School of Gerontology. It lists programs and businesses that perform modifications and repairs to help individuals safely live at home.

www.homemods.org/national-directory

LEGAL

American Bar Association (ABA) – Commission on Law and Aging

The ABA Commission on Law and Aging protects the legal rights, dignity, autonomy, quality of life, and quality of care of older adults through research, policy development, advocacy, education, training, and assistance to lawyers, bar associations and others working on aging issues.

www.americanbar.org/groups/law_aging

Center for Elders and the Courts (CEC)

The CEC serves as the primary resource for the judiciary and court management on aging-related issues. Their efforts include providing training tools, resources, and information to improve court responses to elder abuse and adult guardianships, as well as developing a collaborative community of judges, court staff, and aging experts.

www.eldersandcourts.org

Elder Justice Coalition

This coalition raises public awareness of elder abuse, neglect, and exploitation through research, articles, and monitoring legislation related to elder justice.

www.elderjusticecoalition.com

Justice in Aging

This organization, supported by a network of attorneys, works to protect the rights of older adults living in poverty by securing access to affordable health care, economic security, and the courts for older adults with limited resources. Their efforts include strengthening vital programs through administrative advocacy, litigation, and training attorneys, advocates, and service providers who work with older people.

www.justiceinaging.org

National Academy of Elder Law Attorneys (NAELA)

NAELA is a nonprofit association dedicated to improving the quality of legal services provided to older adults and people with disabilities. Its members consist of attorneys who specialize in solving the legal challenges faced by older Americans and individuals with disabilities. The organization also offers consumer resources and a searchable database of attorneys specializing in elder law and related fields.

www.naela.org

LGBTQ+

Old Lesbians Organizing for Change (OLOC)

This national network works to challenge ageism within their communities and within society at large while promoting the visibility of older lesbians. OLOC achieves this by leading workshops on ageism and collaborating with affiliates and supporters to educate and motivate them about ageism and its effects on everyone.

www.oloc.org

Prime Timers Worldwide (PTWW)

A social organization for adults who self-identify as gay, bisexual, or transgender men, Prime Timers has chapters nationwide. Members engage in their community through volunteering, arts and entertainment activities, participation in support groups, and collaboration with other organizations to raise awareness about gay issues and medical issues.

www.theprimetimersww.com

SAGE – Advocacy & Services for LGBTQ+ Elders

This is a national advocacy and services organization with affiliates across the country focused on addressing issues faced by LGBTQ+ older adults. It builds welcoming communities by providing resources, centers, and programs that support the needs of LGBTQ+ older adults, training those who work with them, and engaging in nationwide advocacy efforts.

www.sageusa.org

National Resource Center on LGBTQ+ Aging

This center, a program of SAGE, is the country's first and only technical assistance resource center engaged in improving the quality of services and support offered to LGBTQ+ older adults, their families, and caregivers. It provides training, technical assistance, and comprehensive educational resources to help this community increase knowledge and awareness about various topics that impact them, such as aging and disability services, elder justice, mental health, allyship, and caregiver support.

www.lgbtagingcenter.org

TRAVEL & RECREATION

Road Scholar

This nonprofit organizes travel learning adventures for lifelong learners worldwide.

www.roadscholar.org

AmeriCorps Seniors

Open to individuals aged fifty-five and older, this branch of AmeriCorps provides service opportunities nationwide through its partner organizations.

www.americorps.gov/serve/americorps-seniors

Senior Planet

Senior Planet is a program created by the national nonprofit organization Older Adults Technology Services (OATS) from AARP. Through this program, OATS helps older adults learn how to use technology to improve their work and lifestyle. It provides on-site training, online courses, and virtual classes on various topics, including fitness.

www.seniorplanet.org

SPECIAL POPULATIONS

Alzheimer's Foundation of America (AFA)

AFA provides support, services, and education to individuals, families, and caregivers affected by Alzheimer's disease and related dementias nationwide. It also funds research to advance treatment and find a cure, and offers professional training, workshops, and educational programs for care providers.

www.alzfdn.org

American Academy of HIV Medicine – HIV & Aging

The American Academy of HIV Medicine has a dedicated page for research, clinical trials, and articles focused on older adults living with HIV.

www.aahivm.org/hiv-and-aging

Americans with Disabilities Act (ADA) National Network

This network provides information, guidance, and training on implementing the Americans with Disabilities Act. The network consists of regional centers, with each center focusing on the unique needs of its cluster of states.

www.adata.org

Alliance for Retired Americans

This is a grassroots advocacy organization working to educate the public and policymakers about critical issues affecting retirees and those planning for retirement. With the help of its members, it advocates and lobbies for related issues such as pensions, prescription drugs, Social Security benefits, Medicaid, and Medicare.

www.retiredamericans.org

Alzheimer's Association

The Alzheimer's Association undertakes various initiatives to accelerate dementia-related advocacy and research, drive risk reduction and early detection, and maximize quality care and support for individuals and families affected by Alzheimer's and dementia. It also provides resources for affected individuals and families, news updates on the latest research and treatments, and information for professionals.

www.alz.org

Helen Keller National Center – Older Adult Program

The HKNC Older Adult Program supports older adults experiencing combined hearing and vision loss, their families, and the professionals who serve them. It accomplishes this through specialized services that provide affected individuals direct access to education, resources, and available benefits.

www.helenkeller.org/hknc/older-adult-program

Michael J. Fox Foundation for Parkinson's Research

This foundation is dedicated to finding a cure for Parkinson's disease through fundraising and supporting research efforts. It also shares information to help those impacted and build awareness about the disease and offers educational resources, including webinars, podcasts, and books.

www.michaeljfox.org

National Alliance on Mental Illness (NAMI)

NAMI is the nation's largest grassroots mental health organization whose mission is to provide advocacy, education, support, and public awareness to help individuals and families affected by mental illness build better lives. Its efforts include providing support groups, a helpline, mental health education, and other resources such as podcasts, webinars, a video resource library, and guides to help those impacted navigate new or challenging experiences.

www.nami.org

National Asian Pacific Center on Aging (NAPCA)

NAPCA promotes the dignity, well-being, and quality of life of older adults of Asian and Pacific Islander descent through programs such as job coaching, senior community service, and dissemination of materials on elder abuse prevention.

www.napca.org

National Caucus & Center on Black Aging, Inc. (NCBA)

The NCBA works to protect and improve the quality of life for minority elderly populations through legislative advocacy, partnerships with like-minded organizations, and employment training.

www.ncba-aging.org

National Council of Certified Dementia Practitioners (NCCDP)

This council provides dementia education, seminars, and certification to health care professionals, first responders, and correctional personnel to ensure proper care for individuals living with dementia.

www.nccdp.org

National Council on Independent Living (NCIL)

NCIL represents thousands of organizations and individuals advocating to enhance the human and civil rights of people with disabilities in the US. Its efforts include training programs, conferences, and policy monitoring.

www.ncil.org

National Federation of the Blind – Seniors Division

The senior branch of this organization is a peer-support group that empowers older adults experiencing vision loss and teaches strategies for independent living. It also provides information about state affiliates, retreats, technology seminars, publications, and other resources on relevant topics.

https://seniors.nfb.org

National Resource Center on HIV and Aging

This center focuses on older adults living with HIV, including long-term survivors. To empower this population to make better health choices, this organization provides information about available supportive services and resources such as webinars, current research data, links to upcoming HIV and aging events, and content on various health management topics.

www.aginghiv.org

Rock Steady Boxing (RSB)

This nonprofit organization is an international network of gyms and health and fitness professionals offering a boxing-inspired program designed for people living with Parkinson's. The non-contact, boxing-based fitness curriculum has been proven to help improve their quality of life and ability to live independently.

www.rocksteadyboxing.org

Women's Institute for a Secure Retirement (WISER)

WISER is a nonprofit organization helping women, educators, and policymakers understand the issues surrounding women's retirement income. Its resources cover topics like Social Security, retirement planning, widowhood, and financial fraud and scams. It also partners with like-minded organizations on various projects, such as educating Latinas and their families about financial challenges in retirement and providing them with the tools and resources needed to help secure their financial future.

www.wiserwomen.org

Us Against Alzheimer's

This nonprofit works to secure more funding for federal research into Alzheimer's and engages in targeted advocacy efforts for minority and youth populations. Its work centers on prevention, early detection and diagnosis, and access to treatments by partnering with the government, scientists, the private sector, and allied organizations.

www.usagainstalzheimers.org

SOME OTHER ALLIES

Last but definitely not least, here are a few other allies to check out. These resources offer services and educational content for living a vibrant life.

The Dementia Guru

Ashley Stevens' educational background in gerontology, along with her graduate certification in dementia care, makes her a powerful advocate in the field. She provides education, resources, and empowerment for caregivers and others impacted by dementia.

www.thedementiaguru.com

Found My Fitness

If you want to dive into the science of nutrition and health, look no further. I first heard Dr. Rhonda Patrick on Joe Rogan's podcast and followed her over to her platform, a treasure trove of information. Her content is both topical and thoroughly researched, offering practical takeaways for people of all ages.

www.foundmyfitness.com

Gero What?!

Christina Peoples brings infectious energy to her work. With an MS in Gerontology and a concentration in aging and business, she creates engaging educational videos, interactive workshops, and other content to explore, educate, and talk about all things aging.

www.gerowhat.com

Next Avenue

A nonprofit, digital journalism publication partnered with the Public Broadcasting System, Next Avenue covers current events, issues, and other topics relevant to older adults.

www.nextavenue.org

The Over 50 Health & Wellness Podcast

Hosted by Kevin English, this podcast is all about active agers living their strongest, healthiest, most fulfilling lives. Listen to inspiring stories of people from all walks of life as they talk about their fitness journeys, along with insights from experts and advocates dedicated to helping older adults thrive.

www.buzzsprout.com/997660

Sixty and Me

This platform provides news articles, videos, expert interviews, and resources on health, wellness, and personal growth to empower and motivate a global readership of women aged sixty and above.

www.sixtyandme.com

NOTES

Introduction

1 Kristie Wilder and Paul Mackun, "While Number of People Age 65 and Older Increased in Almost All Metro Areas, Young Population Declined in Many Metro Areas from 2020 to 2023," United States Census Bureau, last modified June 27, 2024, www.census.gov/library/stories/2024/06/metro-areas-population-age.html. See also, www.census.gov/data/data-tools/quickfacts.html.

2 Alexandre Kalache and Ilona Kickbusch, "A Global Strategy for Healthy Ageing," *World Health* 50, no. 4 (1997): 5, https://iris.who.int/handle/10665/330616.

3 Elizabeth R. Burns, Yara K. Haddad, and Erin M. Parker, "Primary Care Providers' Discussion of Fall Prevention Approaches with Their Older Adult Patients—DocStyles, 2014," *Preventive Medicine Reports* 9, (2018): 149–52, https://doi.org/10.1016/j.pmedr.2018.01.016.

4 MPH Online Program, Baylor University, "Mobility Loss Puts Older Adults at Risk: Research Shows Exercise Can Help," *Age Well Senior Fitness* (blog) November 6, 2019, https://agewellseniorfitness.com/mobility-loss-puts-older-adults-at-risk-research-shows-exercise-can-help/.

5 "Mobility Loss Puts Older Adults at Risk," MPH Online Program, Baylor University.

Chapter 1. The Joy of Movement

1 Sally Goddard Blythe, *The Well Balanced Child: Movement and Early Learning* (Hawthorn Press, 2005), 6–7.

2 Pressing Reset: Restoring the Body Through Movement, the Workshop, version 3.0 (Original Strength, 2017).

Chapter 3. Really . . . How Fit Do I Need to Be?

1 Kalache and Kickbusch, "Global Strategy for Healthy Ageing."

Chapter 4. Don't Neglect Strength and Balance Training

1 *Merriam-Webster Dictionary*, "atrophy," last modified January 14, 2025, www.merriam-webster.com/dictionary/atrophy.

2 Jennifer E. Layne and Miriam E. Nelson, "The Effects of Progressive Resistance Training on Bone Density: A Review," *Medicine & Science in Sports & Exercise* 31, no. 1 (1999): 25–30, https://doi.org/10.1097/00005768 -199901000-00006.

3 Michael Schwenk, Ronny Bergquist, Elisabeth Boulton, Jeanine M. Van Ancum, Corinna Nerz, Michaela Weber et al., "The Adapted Lifestyle-Integrated Functional Exercise Program for Preventing Functional Decline in Young Seniors: Development and Initial Evaluation," *Gerontology* 65, no. 4 (2019): 362–74, https://doi.org/10.1159/000499962.

4 Jonathan M. Sullivan and Andy Baker, *The Barbell Prescription: Strength Training for Life After 40* (The Aasgaard Company, 2016), 61.

5 Sullivan and Baker, *Barbell Prescription*.

Chapter 7. Practice Makes Better

1 Terry Gross, host, *Fresh Air*, podcast, "To 'Keep Sharp' This Year, Keep Learning, Advises Neurosurgeon Sanjay Gupta," NPR, January 4, 2021, www.npr.org/sections/health-shots/2021/01/04/953188905/to-keep -sharp-this-year-keep-learning-advises-neurosurgeon-sanjay-gupta.

2   Renee Montagne, host, *Morning Edition*, podcast, "Learning a New Skill Works Best to Keep Your Brain Sharp," NPR, May 5, 2014, www.npr.org /transcripts/309006780.

3   Lauren Silverman, "Learning a New Skill Works Best to Keep Your Brain Sharp," Morning Edition, *NPR* (blog), May 5, 2014, www.npr.org/sections /health-shots/2014/05/05/309006780/learning-a-new-skill-works-best -to-keep-your-brain-sharp.

4   Kirk I. Erickson, Michelle W. Voss, Ruchika Shaurya Prakash, Chandra-mallika Basak, Amanda Szabo, Laura Chaddock et al., "Exercise Training Increases Size of Hippocampus and Improves Memory," *Proceedings of the National Academy of Sciences of the United States of America* 108, no. 7 (2011): 3017–22, https://doi.org/10.1073/pnas.1015950108.

5   Montagne, "Learning a New Skill."

Chapter 8. Fall Prevention 101

1   Gwen Bergen, Mark R. Stevens, and Elizabeth R. Burns, "Falls and Fall Injuries Among Adults Aged ≥65 Years—United States, 2014," *Morbidity and Mortality Weekly Report* 65, no. 37 (2016): 993–98, https://doi.org /10.15585/mmwr.mm6537a2.

2   Jacqueline Crockford, "6 Exercises to Improve Agility," American Council on Exercise, March 19, 2014, www.acefitness.org/education-and-resources /professional/expert-articles/3782/6-exercises-to-improve-agility.

3   Nicole Thompson, "Joint Mobility and Stability," American Council on Exercise, March 7, 2019, www.acefitness.org/fitness-certifications/ace -answers/exam-preparation-blog/1189/joint-mobility-and-stability.

4   Jane E. Brody, "Hearing Loss Threatens Mind, Life and Limb," *New York Times*, December 31, 2018, www.nytimes.com/2018/12/31/well/live/hearing -loss-threatens-mind-life-and-limb.html.

5   "Hearing Loss Linked to Threefold Risk of Falling," *JHU Gazette*, March 5, 2012, https://gazette.jhu.edu/2012/03/05/hearing-loss-linked-to -threefold-risk-of-falling/.

6   "Hearing Loss," *JHU Gazette*.

7   Stephen R. Lord and Julia Dayhew, "Visual Risk Factors for Falls in Older People," *Journal of the American Geriatrics Society* 49, no. 5 (2001): 508–15, https://doi.org/10.1046/j.1532-5415.2001.49107.x.

8   Lord and Dayhew, "Visual Risk Factors."

9   Arunima Awale, Thomas J. Hagedorn, Alyssa B. Dufour, Hylton B. Menz, Virginia A. Casey, and Marian T. Hannan, "Foot Function, Foot Pain, and Falls in Older Adults: The Framingham Foot Study," *Gerontology* 63, no. 4 (2017): 318–24, https://pmc.ncbi.nlm.nih.gov/articles/PMC5501294/.

10 Awale et al., "Foot Function."

11 Luisa Torres, "Simple Ways to Prevent Falls in Older Adults," *Weekend Edition Sunday*, NPR, July 14, 2019, www.npr.org/sections/health-shots/2019/07/14/741310765/simple-ways-to-prevent-falls-in-older-adults.

Chapter 9. The Branches of Our Physical Function

1   Pete McCall, "Stability vs. Mobility: What's the Difference?," American Council on Exercise, February 5, 2018, www.acefitness.org/education-and-resources/professional/expert-articles/6928/stability-vs-mobility-what-s-the-difference/.

2   McCall, "Stability vs. Mobility."

3   Eduardo Cadore, Ronei Silveira Pinto, Martim Bottaro, and Mikel Izquierdo, "Strength and Endurance Training Prescription in Healthy and Frail Elderly," *Aging and Disease* 5, no. 3 (2014): 183–95, https://doi.org/10.14336/AD.2014.0500183.

4   Sullivan and Baker, *Barbell Prescription*.

Chapter 10. The Mental Aspect of Movement

1   Cody Sipe, "Exercise for Optimal Brain Function," American Council on Exercise, September 22, 2017, www.acefitness.org/education-and-resources/professional/expert-articles/6570/exercise-for-optimal-brain-function/.

2   Fernando Gomez-Pinilla and Charles Hillman, "The Influence of Exercise on Cognitive Abilities," *Comprehensive Physiology* 3, no. 1 (2013): 403–28, https://pmc.ncbi.nlm.nih.gov/articles/PMC3951958/.

3   "Cognitive Health and Older Adults," National Institute on Aging, last modified June 11, 2024, www.nia.nih.gov/health/cognitive-health-and -older-adults.

4   Gomez-Pinilla and Hillman, "Influence of Exercise."

Chapter 12. Move for Life

1   J. Eric Ahlskog, Yonas E. Geda, Neill R. Graff-Radford, and Ronald C. Petersen, "Physical Exercise as a Preventive or Disease-Modifying Treatment of Dementia and Brain Aging," *Mayo Clinic Proceedings* 86, no. 9 (2011): 876–84, https://doi.org/10.4065/mcp.2011.0252.

INDEX

ABOUT
THE AUTHOR

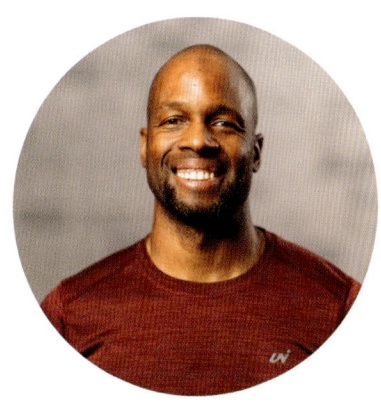

Damien A. Joyner is a health coach with UC San Diego's WorkStrong Program, where he helps UC employees recover from workplace injuries, return to work pain-free, and graduate with personalized exercise and training plans. Based in San Diego, he also specializes in working with individuals aged fifty and older through his business, Incremental Fitness™. His approach incorporates balance training, strength training, and functional movement.

After earning his Juris Doctor, Damien transitioned to the fitness industry in 2016. He gained experience with the general population before specializing in active aging. His background includes leading group classes for San Diego's Feeling Fit Club, working as a fitness specialist at Golden Door Wellness Resort, and speaking for the Fall Prevention Speaker's Bureau.

As a subject matter expert for the American Council on Exercise (ACE), Damien serves on the Virtual Certification Committee and Certification Advisory Board (CAB). In this role, he has also contributed to video study materials, participated as a panelist in ACE's virtual press conference on Exercise and Brain Health for Older Adults, led the webinar "Exercise Strategies for Clients with Physically Demanding Jobs," and featured in AARP, SilverSneakers®, *EatingWell*®, and *Fit&Well* publications.

Damien is passionate about improving his clients' quality of life and promoting mental and physical well-being through self-care. In his free time, he enjoys exploring San Francisco on foot, hiking the Grand Canyon, discovering new music, and appreciating sunrises and hummingbirds. Connect with him at incrementalfit.com and on Instagram @damien.a.joyner.

ABOUT NORTH ATLANTIC BOOKS

North Atlantic Books (NAB) is an independent, nonprofit publisher committed to a bold exploration of the relationships between mind, body, spirit, and nature. Founded in 1974, NAB aims to nurture a holistic view of the arts, sciences, humanities, and healing. To make a donation or to learn more about our books, authors, events, and newsletter, please visit www.northatlantic books.com.